Fundamentals of Research Methodology for Healthcare Professionals

Fifth edition

Hilla Brink

Gisela van Rensburg

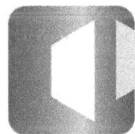

juta

Fundamentals of Research Methodology
for Healthcare Professionals

First published 1996
Second edition 2006
Third edition 2012
Fourth edition 2018
Fifth edition 2022

Juta and Company (Pty) Ltd
First Floor, Sunclare Building, 21 Dreyer Street, Claremont, 7708
PO Box 14373, Lansdowne 7779, Cape Town, South Africa
www.juta.co.za

© 2022 Juta and Company (Pty) Ltd

ISBN 978 1 48513 168 7 (Print)
ISBN 978 1 48513 169 4 (WebPDF)

Acknowledgment:
The Author and Publisher wish to acknowledge the contribution of Christa van der Walt
to previous editions.

Project Specialist: Fuzlin Toffar
Editor: Rod Prodgers
Proofreader: Linda van de Vijver
Cover Designer: Renaissance Studio
Typesetter: LT Design Worx
Indexer: Language Mechanics

Typeset in Minion Pro 10.5pt on 13pt

Preface

Fundamentals of Research Methodology for Healthcare Professionals (5th edition) is intended specifically for healthcare professionals and undergraduate students who are introduced to research as a new way of experiencing reality. The book's major purpose is to provide information about the logic of scientific enquiry generally, to guide novice researchers through the research process, and to stimulate awareness of the myriad researchable and research-needed questions encountered in daily practice. The readers are introduced to a unique language, new rules and new experiences in such a way that it will assist them in expanding their perceptions and methods of reasoning. This text is not intended to be a comprehensive, in-depth source that provides all the answers relating to the research process; it should be seen, rather, as a stepping stone to more sophisticated textbooks and as facilitating entry into and understanding of the 'research world' and its contribution to the delivery of quality healthcare. It emphasises using and applying research, and provides conceptual and non-technical descriptions of the methods used by researchers. It not only covers the steps of the research process, but also explains what a researcher does, while serving as a guide to evaluating each of the steps in the research process. The inclusion of practical examples is intended to make the text more understandable. Both qualitative and quantitative approaches are used and are presented and illustrated with examples from practice. Each chapter contains outcomes, examples, summaries and exercises specific to the chapter content, in order to facilitate understanding and assimilation of the information provided. An extensive glossary is provided to assist the reader in evaluating research reports and in becoming acquainted with the terminology used in the text. As all healthcare professionals' research roles are to contribute to the development of evidence-based practice, we trust that this new edition will continue to be an invaluable source to novice researchers. The book is fundamentally grounded in the belief that research is an intellectually and professionally rewarding field, and that developing research skills and creating a research culture are critical to the health sciences. The aim of this book is to facilitate understanding and stimulate curiosity and interest in research.

Gisela van Rensburg
September 2022

Contents

Preface.. iii

About the authors xi

CHAPTER 1

Orientation to health sciences research 1

What is research? 2

Definitions of research 3

What is health sciences research? 4

Ways of acquiring knowledge 4

Tradition 5

Authorities 5

Logical reasoning 6

Experience 7

Trial and error 7

Intuition 7

Borrowing 7

The scientific method 8

Limitations of the scientific method 9

Main types of scientific research 10

Reasons for conducting health sciences research 11

Roles of healthcare professionals in research 12

Using research knowledge to promote evidence-based practice 13

The hierarchy of evidence 14

Systematic, integrative and scoping reviews 16

CHAPTER 2

Research and theory 19

The nature of scientific theory 19

Definitions of theory 20

Types of theory 20

Theory-related terms 22

Development of theory 27

Testing of theory 30

The relationship between theory and research 30

CHAPTER 3

Ethical considerations in the conduct of health sciences research 33

Codes of ethical research 34

Fundamental ethical principles 35
    Principle of respect for persons/human dignity 35
    Principle of beneficence 37
    Principle of justice 38
Procedures and mechanisms for protecting human rights 39
    Informed consent 39
    Issues relating to informed consent 42
    The risk–benefit ratio 43
    Scientific honesty and other responsibilities 44
    Ethics review boards and committees 45
Evaluation of the ethical elements of a research proposal or report 46

CHAPTER 4
An overview of the research process 49
The research process 49
Major phases and steps in the research process 51
    Phase 1: The conceptual phase 51
    Phase 2: The empirical phase 54
    Phase 3: The interpretive phase 55
    Phase 4: The communication phase 55
Other models of the research process 56
    Model using five steps 57
    Model using eight steps 57
Research setting 57

CHAPTER 5
Selecting or identifying research problems 59
What is a research topic? 59
Research problem and purpose 60
    Origins of research problems 61
    Considerations regarding research problems 63

CHAPTER 6
The literature review 69
Definitions 69
Purpose of the literature review 70
Types of information and sources 72
    1. Facts, statistics and research findings 72
    2. Theories or interpretations 72
    3. Methods and procedures 72
    4. Opinions, beliefs or points of view 73
    5. Anecdotes, clinical impressions or narrations of incidents and
       situations 73

Primary and secondary sources.. 73
Depth and breadth of the review.. 74
Developing a search strategy 74
   Using libraries and electronic databases.......................... 74
   Identifying sources.. 75
   Locating sources.. 76
   Compiling lists of identified sources and searching for them........ 76
The review process 76
   Systematically recording references................................. 77
   Determining additional ways of locating sources 78
   Reading sources critically... 78
   Writing the review report 78
   Evaluating the research review 80

CHAPTER 7

Refining and defining the research question 83
Refining the research question 83
Research questions.. 85
   Example 7.1... 85
   Example 7.2... 85
Research hypotheses 86
   Types of hypotheses.. 88
   Formulating hypotheses 89
Research aims and objectives.. 90
   Example 7.3... 90
Identifying variables 91
   Types of variables 91
   Defining variables 92
Research proposal... 94

CHAPTER 8

Quantitative research... 99
Important concepts and principles in quantitative research
designs... 100
   Rigour 100
   Causality... 100
   Probability 101
   Bias 101
   Triangulation.. 102
Basic and applied research 102
Time dimension in research 103
Classification of research designs 105

Experimental designs 106
Non-experimental designs 113
Epidemiological research 117
Epidemiological process 118
Evaluating quantitative research designs 119

CHAPTER 9

Qualitative research designs and introduction to mixed methods research 121
Overview of qualitative research 122
Searching the literature in qualitative research 123
Phenomenology 124
Ethnography 126
Grounded theory 127
Philosophical inquiry 128
Rigour in qualitative research 129
Choice of research design 132
An introduction to mixed methods research 133
Major types of mixed methods designs 134

CHAPTER 10

Sampling 139
Basic sampling concepts 139
Population 140
Sampling frame 141
Parameter and statistics 141
A representative sample 141
Sampling error 142
Sampling bias 142
Sampling approaches 143
Probability or random sampling 143
Non-probability sampling 148
Sample choice 153
Sample adequacy 155

CHAPTER 11

Data collection 157
The data-collection process 157
What data will be collected? 158
How will data be collected? 159
Who will collect the data? 160
Where will the data be collected? 160
When will the data be collected? 160
Data-collection methods 160

Observation 160
Self-report techniques 162
Physiological measures 171
Other techniques 172

CHAPTER 12

Data quality... 175
Types of error 175
Random errors.. 175
Systematic errors 176
Sources of measurement error 176
Participant factors 176
Researcher factors 177
Environmental factors 177
Instrumentation factors 177
Validity of data-collection instruments 177
Content validity 177
Face validity 178
Criterion-related validity 178
Construct validity 180
Validity of qualitative data 181
Reliability of data-collection instruments 181
Stability 182
Internal consistency... 182
Equivalence reliability.. 182
Relationship between reliability and validity........................ 183
Trustworthiness 183
Data enhancement strategies organised by phase of the study 186
Other factors affecting data quality 186
Sensitivity... 187
Efficiency... 187
Appropriateness 187
Ability to generalise 187
The pilot study and pre-test.. 187
Measurement evaluation 188

CHAPTER 13

Data analysis 191
Analysis of quantitative data 192
Choosing appropriate statistical procedures 193
Descriptive statistics.. 193
Inferential statistics... 203
Use of graphics.. 205

Interpretation of quantitative data.. 206
Analysis of qualitative data.. 206
Data-analysis evaluation.. 208
Protection of data in the online space.. 209

CHAPTER 14
Research reports and report evaluation 213
   Purpose of a research report.. 213
   Report formats 214
   Planning the report... 214
   Structure of the report 216
      The title.. 216
      Abstract 217
      Introduction to the study 217
      Literature review 217
      Research methodology... 218
      Research design and strategy 218
      Participants.. 218
      Instrument and data collection 218
      Data analysis 219
      Results or findings.. 219
      Discussion 219
      References... 220
   Style of the report 220
   Technical layout of the report 221
   The ethics of report writing 222
   Critical evaluation of the report 222
   Productive writing... 223

Bibliography 227
Glossary 237
Index.. 249

About the authors

The late Professor **Hilla Brink**, formerly attached to the Department of Health Studies at the University of South Africa (Unisa), was a nurse scholar of international repute and an acknowledged nurse educator, nursing and health researcher, and academic. The first edition of this book filled a serious gap in undergraduate academic literature in nursing at the time. The later editions of *Fundamentals of Research Methodology for Healthcare Professionals* were greatly appreciated by the allied health sciences for their clarity and simplicity. Hilla Brink will always be remembered by colleagues for the way in which she could explain the most complex concepts in plain, understandable terms – an acquired gift of the true scholar.

Gisela van Rensburg obtained her DLit et Phil at the University of South Africa (Unisa). She is a Professor in the Department of Health Studies at Unisa. She is actively involved in the supervision of Masters and doctoral students. Gisela is engaged in a variety of projects on research capacity development and the teaching of research methodology. Her research focus is on health sciences education and reflective practice. Her clinical interests are in orthopaedic nursing and the psycho-social aspects of HIV and Aids. She has been involved in a number of national and international research projects in these fields.

Orientation to health sciences research

LEARNING OUTCOMES

On completion of this chapter, you should be able to demonstrate your understanding of:

- research, and health sciences research
- ways of acquiring knowledge
- the scientific method of inquiry
- the main types of health sciences research
- the differences between the major features of qualitative and quantitative research
- the differences and similarities between the research and problem-solving processes
- reasons for conducting health sciences research
- the various roles of healthcare professionals in research
- evidence-based practice

We have become familiar with the term 'research' in our everyday lives. We have become part of research, knowingly or unknowingly. Surveys are conducted on street corners or by counting vehicles or driving patterns. Short opinion polls are used on social media such as Facebook to determine likes and dislikes of a product. We are presented with findings of studies in newspapers or on television. At times one regards these findings as obvious information and unnecessary. During a pandemic such as Covid-19, the findings of clinical trials are used to provide the necessary motivation and justification for vaccination. Some findings of research studies are received with great appreciation and understanding whereas in other instances they are regarded with apprehension and suspicion. Nevertheless, research is an integral part of everyday life.

In any profession one asks questions about what one is doing and how one does it. These meaningful questions lead to research (Ellis, 2022). Research is therefore important in any profession. Professionals need knowledge on which to base their practice, and scientific knowledge provides a particularly solid foundation. Professionals also need specialised knowledge and tools to work effectively, and their inability to meet research challenges may become a critical factor in determining the viability of their professions.

Research is thus an integral part of healthcare practice, education and management. Accordingly, 'research-mindedness' should be fostered in healthcare professionals from the start of their training. They need to be aware of, and knowledgeable about, the application of research in their practice. This awareness must be reflected in evidence-based practice and evidence-informed decision-making.

This book intends to orientate you in the field of health sciences research and to equip you with fundamental research tools and skills. It will also assist you in becoming both an enthusiastic researcher and a critical consumer of research findings in day-to-day practice.

What is research?

The term 'research' attracts such an array of definitions that we often accept them without considering exactly what they mean. In the vernacular, the term signifies almost any sort of information-gathering or checking. Such activity is not, however, aligned to definitions accepted by the scientific community. Leedy and Ormrod (2010) caution that research should not merely refer to information-gathering, digging or the transference of facts from one source to another. In science, research refers to the exploration, discovery and careful study of unexplained phenomena. It entails a systematic and credible way of finding answers to questions, solutions to problems, of generating new ideas or confirming existing knowledge (Harvey & Land, 2021).

In this book the term 'research in the health sciences' is used to signify the scientific approach to research. However, you will encounter a variety of definitions of scientific research. Within these definitions we identify the following characteristics:

- Research results in an **increase in knowledge**, which in turn contributes to an existing body of knowledge. The ultimate aim of research in the health sciences is to provide strong evidence on which the practice of quality care can be based (Burns & Grove, 2020).
- Research starts with a **question** or a **problem**.
- Knowledge is obtained by means of at least one of the following methods: search, **discovery** or **inquiry**. This implies that the researcher is actively involved in looking for information which is not readily available or for which there is no generally accepted evidence.
- The search is **systematic** and **diligent**. It involves planning, organisation and persistence. The researcher proceeds in an orderly manner, according to a logical, predetermined scheme, and tries to minimise the likelihood of results being influenced by faults in the apparatus, in their methodology or by their expectations (Grove, Gray & Burns, 2018; Harvey & Land, 2021).
- Research is a **process**. It implies a purpose, a series of actions and a goal. The purpose gives the process direction, and the actions are organised into steps to achieve the goal. Research thus constitutes a series of planned actions rather than haphazard ones.
- Research is a **scientific process**. It is the systematic application of the scientific method. Science as a process implies orderly, logical and public activity. 'Public' in this

context means that research findings, and the methods used to acquire them, are made known to members of the research community. The researcher must, therefore, record every step in the process in detail to enable others to evaluate and repeat the inquiry in different contexts. Inasmuch as the scientific process implies precision, accuracy and a lack of bias, it also involves scepticism. Unconfirmed observations, propositions or statements – even when made by an authority on a subject – are open to refute and analysis and need to be confirmed. Researchers must, therefore, provide evidence or logical justification in support of their conclusions or statements of fact, so that these can be scrutinised. Though it is impossible for researchers to exert total control, the scientific method nevertheless implies that they should attempt to exercise as much control as possible over the research situation to increase the reliability and validity of the findings.

Definitions of research

- 'a systematic process of collecting, analysing and interpreting information in order to increase our understanding of phenomena of interest' (Leedy & Ormrod, 2010: 2)
- '[a] systematic inquiry that uses disciplined methods to answer questions or solve problems. The ultimate goal of research is to develop and expand knowledge' (Polit & Beck, 2021: 2).

Research is usually divided into two categories: quantitative and qualitative research. The former focuses on measurable aspects of human behaviour, while the latter concentrates on aspects such as meaning, experience and understanding.

Quantitative research is characterised by the following principles:
1. Adopting a concise and narrow focus
2. Accepting preconceived theories about concepts' interrelation
3. Gathering evidence that is rooted in objective reality
4. Collecting data under controlled conditions
5. Reporting the data in a way that focuses on relatively few concepts.

Qualitative research is characterised by the following principles:
1. Accepting multiple realities
2. Being committed to identifying an approach which supports the research
3. Remaining committed to participants' perspectives
4. Conducting the study in a way that limits the disruption of a phenomenon's natural context
5. Reporting the data in a way that supports participant commentaries.

A researcher's choice of design ultimately depends upon the research problem. Despite the apparent distinctions between the quantitative and qualitative approaches, combinations are possible, valid and sometimes required. Researchers nowadays refer to mixed methods research, where quantitative and qualitative methods are used, as a third approach. Mixed methods designs include at least one quantitative and one qualitative method that embrace incompatible assumptions about the nature of the world and allow researchers to mix epistemologies. The question one would typically ask is whether mixing methods will add more value to a study than one single method. More information on mixed methods will be provided later in the book.

What is health sciences research?

Research in the health sciences is multidimensional. It is concerned with clinical research, education, management, ethics, legislation and many other aspects. It is a systematic process of inquiry designed to generate trustworthy evidence in the realms of practice, education, administration and informatics.

Bowling and Ebrahim (2005) and Ellis (2019) argue that healthcare professionals are committed to evidence-informed care that enhances the following:

- **Effectiveness:** the ability of an intervention to work for everyone who may need it
- **Efficacy:** whether an intervention helps a specific group of people in which it is tested
- **Efficiency:** whether the intervention/treatment is also cost-effective
- **Equity:** whether healthcare is available to everyone
- **Acceptability:** whether intervention/treatment is acceptable to the patients, with emphasis on patient choice, patient-centred care and community empowerment
- **Implementation:** monitoring and evaluating change.

Researchers' divergent opinions and preferences on how to conduct research do not affect the term's definition. The same rules of the scientific method apply to the research process as do the logical steps. Research is conducted through a structured and conscious application of a scientific method to the exploration of a topic of interest in order to understand the topic better or to establish new truths about the topic. The researcher's goal is the development of a prevailing knowledge base. Indeed, healthcare debates tend to stem from legitimate investigative subjects within the discipline.

Ways of acquiring knowledge

In addition to being an essential element of research, the scientific method is also one of the most reliable methods of knowledge acquisition. Acquiring knowledge through scientific methods is the notion of discovering new things using the senses and, in the case of research, using different methods. Research is, however, only one source. This has been acknowledged by healthcare professionals, and they have come to rely on several sources to inform their practice. Healthcare professionals may be uncertain about the sources of information for a variety of reasons. The nature of education and experiences in life and the healthcare field may lead to preconceived ideas, lack of confidence, repetitive practices or suspicion of research. In some instances, research is regarded as being a threat to the values in healthcare, traditional healthcare knowledge and so-called 'proven' ways of working, and could be regarded as being imposed by researchers on practitioners or clinicians. Such perceptions may affect evidence-based practice (EBP). An integrative review conducted in 2016 indicated that participants (nurses) acknowledged that they did not always use best evidence to support their practice, although they displayed a positive approach to research and EBP (Saunders & Vehviläinen-Julkunen, 2016). In an attempt to demystify research, one also has to understand the different ways of knowing.

Tradition

Traditions have been handed down from one generation to the next. For many decades a traditional stance regarding healthcare was that years of experience was the key to excellent thinking and care and was enough to make decisions about a patient or patient care (Harvey & Land, 2021). Knowledge can also be handed down from one generation to the next, and often leads to the belief that certain actions are performed simply because 'they have always been done that way'. Although tradition is not necessarily based on evidence, it has certain advantages. Individual researchers need not start anew to understand the world or a particular phenomenon. Tradition facilitates communication because it provides a common frame of reference for each member of an investigative group. However, tradition also poses some problems. Many traditions have never been evaluated for validity. They may also contribute to stagnation of practice, instead of encouraging innovation. This leads to a ritualisation of practice, in which the basis becomes inflexible and developments in the field are rejected without examination (Polit & Beck, 2021).

Harvey and Land (2021) explain an example of tradition versus research which refers to anti-thrombolytic therapy ('clot-busting' drugs). These authors refer to an analysis of several randomised controlled trials during the early 1990s which established that a reduction in mortality rates by approximately 20% was achievable using anti-thrombolytic therapy. In 14 further reviews of similar research no mention was made of the treatment nor was it reported that the treatment was still experimental. This disagreement among researchers resulted in a total of 25 years passing before anti-thrombolytic therapy was introduced as a routine treatment, saving numerous lives. During this period many lives would have been saved if the therapy had been adopted earlier.

Authorities

Authorities offer specialised expertise, experience or power and are able to influence opinions and behaviours. Governmental and institutional structures, along with statutory research healthcare bodies, establish policies and procedures that dictate the practices of healthcare professionals. Such reliance on authorities is, to some extent, inevitable because we cannot all become experts on every problem we encounter.

However, while authorities are rarely questioned, they do have certain limitations as an information source. Authorities often build their knowledge around personal experience and engage in practices which are seldom challenged (Polit & Beck, 2021). As a result, the statements of one authority may be contradicted or refuted by another equally prestigious authority. Authorities may pick their favourite opinions, treatments or practices based on certain literature and ignore others. How can we resolve the conflicting claims? In practice, unless we can find objective and acceptable criteria for resolution, there will be ongoing disputes, slanderous commentary or even aggressive behaviour. Therefore, certain 'rules' must be used to interpret the literature to support treatment. EBP guides us to move from opinion-based decision-making to evidence-based decision-making. An example of acquiring knowledge through authority could be the banning of tobacco product sales as one of the Covid-19 regulations early in the pandemic. This ban did not seem to be supported by evidence or science-based information.

Logical reasoning

Burns and Grove (2020) point out that the researcher may select an inductive or a deductive stance, or a combination of both, depending on the nature of the research being conducted. While each provides a useful means of understanding and organising phenomena, and plays an important role in scientific research, neither is without limitations when used as a sole basis of knowledge.

Inductive reasoning involves developing generalisations from specific observations. The researcher obtains information through observation and makes generalisations based upon them. For example, a physiotherapist observes that certain patients in a spinal ward seem to be more anxious than others. Through discussions, she discovers that the anxious patients have little knowledge about their medical conditions, the implications and expected outcomes, whereas the calmer patients are aware of what their conditions involve. Using inductive reasoning, she concludes that a lack of understanding of one's condition contributes to a high degree of anxiety.

The disadvantage of inductive reasoning is that the knowledge arrived at is highly dependent on the representativeness of the samples obtained. The reasoning process offers no mechanism for criterion evaluation and no built-in checks for determining the validity of a conclusion. If the initial observations and/or conclusion prove false, more questions may arise.

Deductive reasoning involves the derivation of specific observations or predictions from general principles. The researcher moves from a general premise to a particular conclusion. For example, if researchers believe that anyone who experiences the loss of a close family member due to complications of the Covid-19 vaccine will be against vaccination, then they may conclude that because Peter Ndou's father has died, he will not want to be vaccinated. Researchers use deductive reasoning to apply a general principle to a specific case.

Deductive reasoning can also lead to erroneous conclusions, however, since a conclusion's validity depends on the correctness of the general premise. Cultural or gender stereotypes provide one example.

Experience

Our experience represents a familiar and functional knowledge source. In some instances, experience and opinions are used to make quick decisions. However, individual experiences may be too restricted to allow for the development of generalisations. Every person experiences or perceives phenomena or occurrences differently, and our experiences tend to be informed by our values and prejudices.

Trial and error

This method is sometimes adopted when a researcher encounters a problem for the first time and intervenes using the most reasonable solution available. If the intervention is successful, they adopt it for future use. If it is not, they try alternative approaches until they find a suitable solution. In a way, the researcher engages in a form of informal experimentation here.

While this method offers a practical means of securing knowledge, it can be both fallible and inefficient. Its haphazardness means that it may not be possible for other researchers to repeat an experiment.

Intuition

Intuition is often the first port of call when one has to make a decision. We therefore sometimes acquire knowledge as sudden insight. Unfortunately, though, intuition does not lend itself to empirical testing. It is generally considered an insufficient means of approaching information within the context of research, but can serve as a guiding and creative addition in some instances.

Borrowing

According to Burns and Grove (2020), 'borrowing' in health sciences involves the appropriation and use of knowledge from other fields or disciplines. Some healthcare sciences have incorporated information from disciplines such as sociology, psychology and education, and successfully applied it directly to their practice. However, borrowing is not necessarily an adequate means of answering questions related to healthcare practice, particularly if researchers do not understand the context from which they borrow ideas, theories or evidence. When information is used out of context, significant distortions of knowledge may result.

The scientific method

The scientific method refers to a set of systematic, disciplined and orderly procedures used to acquire information.

Table 1.1 summarises the differences between the scientific method and other methods of knowledge acquisition.

Table 1.1 Differences between the scientific method and other methods of knowledge acquisition

The scientific method	Alternative methods
● Uses empirical inquiry (data are collected by means of observation via the human senses and/or measuring instruments)	● May accept inflated explanations, based on opinions and not research-informed evidence: a sales representative of prosthetics may argue that 'most patients do exceptionally well after a knee replacement'
● Uses a systematic approach (i e the researcher moves in an orderly fashion through a series of steps according to a predetermined plan of action): in her motivation for a new generation ventilator for pre-term babies, the unit manager of the NICU refers to the findings of a recently published systematic review	● The unit manager of a NICU refers to a discussion she had with a friend who works at another hospital that recently bought a specific ventilator. She is very positive about it. Although the information was practical and valuable, her motivation was a bit haphazard and unsystematic. On questions from a Hospital Board member as to whether she has any research evidence to support her motivation and what the cost will be, she said she will need to come back to the Board with that information. Her request was unsuccessful and minuted to be followed up
● Makes empirical data public (i e all steps and findings are recorded precisely and in an unbiased manner and published or presented to fellow researchers so that they can be checked and verified)	● Are frequently not recorded or documented or shared in other ways
● Uses control and objectivity (i e the investigator uses checks and mechanisms to minimise the possibility of biases and confounding factors)	● Make little or no attempt to control variables
● Strives for the development of conceptual explanations or theories	● Select evidence from personal experiences or performances

⁀▶

The scientific method	Alternative methods
● Strives for generalisability	● Often focus on isolated events
● Tends not to deal with metaphysical explanations that cannot be empirically tested	● May be highly metaphysical or spiritual
● Uses tested reasoning (verification and falsification) or justification	● Are frequently based on rituals

Limitations of the scientific method

The scientific community differs in their perceptions and understanding of what 'science' means. While some scientists have rigid views, others are more relativistic. Generally, though, it is accepted that science is changing all the time, and that what we refer to as 'knowledge' is provisional and based on the best current research. It is thus imperative that before embarking on a new research project, researchers take into account current advances in their discipline as well as the accepted methods of investigation.

Traditionally, some theorists held that the scientist and the object of study were separate, and that the object was governed by laws and rules which do not vary. Accordingly, the scientists' views and values were believed to be uninfluenced by their discoveries.

Qualitative researchers have responded to these arguments by labelling the 'traditional' scientific approach as reductionist, implying traditionalists would rather focus on studying a disease than studying the person living with the disease. Qualitative researchers believe that the above approach is an insufficient means of capturing the complexities of the human experience as it focuses on a few concepts rather than the broader meaning. It also inadequately answers moral or value-laden questions and tends to ignore the fact that human behaviour is too complex to be measured by conventional scientific instruments (Polit & Beck, 2021). Quantitative researchers move systematically through the research process by using a series of steps according to a prespecified plan. The methods are designed to control the research situation with the aim of minimising bias and maximising validity.

Indeed, scientists have increasingly begun to acknowledge that their findings may be influenced by their own values and perspectives, and that this cannot (and should not) be ignored or eliminated for the convenience of research. Although they strive to be objective, scientists now recognise that these factors may never be entirely eradicated and believe them to be symptomatic of the humanistic and holistic philosophies they hold (Burns & Grove, 2020).

Main types of scientific research

Research can be categorised according to perspective and purpose. Burns and Grove (2019) point out that the distinction between applied and basic (or pure) research depends on the researcher's aim. When researchers seek to develop theories that increase knowledge, they will engage in basic research. When they aim to solve problems, or make decisions for practical purposes, they conduct applied research. Gray (2021) explains the purpose of basic and applied research as follows:

- Basic research expands knowledge of social or organisational processes, whereas applied research improves the understanding of specific social or organisational problems.
- Basic research develops universal principles, whereas applied research creates solutions to social or organisational problems.
- Basic research produces findings of significance and value to society, whereas applied research develops findings of practical relevance to public and organisational stakeholders.

Research can also be classified according to two categories: experimental and non-experimental. In experimental research an intervention or treatment is actively introduced. Such studies are called clinical trials or randomised control trials. In these studies, the researcher is an active agent in the study. In non-experimental research the researchers are 'bystanders' or observers, therefore collecting data without intervening.

Experimental designs are further divided into two sub-types: the true experiment and the quasi-experiment.

The true **experimental approach** has three main characteristics:

- **Manipulation of the independent variable.** Manipulation involves the researcher doing something to study the participants. The independent variable is manipulated by, for example, administering a treatment or intervention to some participants or groups and not to others; or by administering alternative treatment or intervention to other participants or groups. The independent variable is therefore varied and then the outcome is observed.
- **Control over the experimental situation.** Controls can include devising counterfactual approximations. The researcher introduces control by, for example, having a control group or using controlled conditions.
- **Randomisation.** Randomisation means that, from a group that was randomly selected from the target population, every research participant has an equal chance of being assigned to either the control group or the experimental group. Therefore, the researcher assigns participants to a control or an experimental condition on a random basis.

The **quasi-experimental** approach lacks both randomisation and control over the experimental situation.

The **non-experimental** approach applies to research where manipulation of the independent variable is not possible and/or where other experimental approaches are impractical or inappropriate. Burns and Grove (2019) and Polit and Beck (2021) suggest the following classifications for this approach:

- **Descriptive designs,** which include both typical and comparative descriptive designs as well as case studies. The purpose of descriptive studies is to observe, describe and document a situation as it naturally occurs and could serve as a point of departure for generating hypotheses or developing theories. Descriptive designs can be correlational or univariate in nature. Descriptive correlational research describes the relationships among variables rather than supporting inferences of causality. Univariate descriptive studies describe the frequency of occurrence of a condition or behaviour, rather than studying relationships. In epidemiological studies descriptive designs are prevalence studies or incidence studies.

  Descriptive designs are categorised according to the sequence in which the data are collected, and include the following:
  - Retrospective (or *ex post facto*) designs measure variables which occurred in the past.
  - Prospective designs measure variables which will occur during the course of research.
  - The timeframe of research dictates whether the design is longitudinal (a design that follows research participants over time) or cross-sectional (a design which examines phenomena that exist during the period of study).

- **Correlational designs.** These designs study the effect of a potential cause that cannot be manipulated, thus examining the relationships between variables. Correlational designs include retrospective designs (eg case-control design), prospective non-experimental designs (cohort design), natural experiments (eg where exposed patients are compared to non-exposed patients) and path analysis (model testing).

Although there are similarities between research and problem-solving, there are also key differences. Their purposes, for example, are quite different. Problem-solving seeks a solution to an immediate problem which exists for an individual (or individuals) in a given setting. The purpose of scientific research is broader: its main aim is to obtain knowledge that can be generalised, making it applicable across a variety of contexts and groups. Furthermore, the research problem must be positioned within the context of existing scholarship and must conform to a theoretical framework.

Reasons for conducting health sciences research

Healthcare professionals need to acknowledge the value of research on which they can base their practice in order to improve the quality of healthcare. Health sciences research is a continuous process and as new treatments are developed, they will need testing against current ones. A sound, robust and transparent scientific process to build evidence is produced incrementally and not on a trial-and-error basis.

Reasons for research include:

- healthcare improvements
- earning and defending a professional status
- establishing scientifically defensible reasons for healthcare practices
- increasing the repertoire of scientifically defensible intervention options
- finding ways to enhance the cost-effectiveness of healthcare services
- providing a base for standard-setting and quality assurance
- providing evidence of weaknesses and strengths within the field
- providing evidence in support of requests for resources
- providing a base for self-correction of misinterpretations and myths (Burns & Grove, 2019).

Roles of healthcare professionals in research

EBP depends on well-informed practitioners. All healthcare professionals are at some stage engaged in research activities along a continuum of participation. On the one side one has 'consumers' of research who read research reports to keep abreast with findings to gain knowledge on a topic that may affect their practice. On the other side of the continuum are the 'producers' of research, those healthcare professionals who actively conduct research. Between the extreme sides of the continuum lies a variety of research activities that are undertaken by healthcare professionals and researchers. While it is possible for a novice researcher to conduct basic studies, a postgraduate degree is required to obtain the status of independent researcher. However, every healthcare professional should at least be involved in the evaluation of research findings. As research consumers, professionals are obliged to become familiar with research findings and to determine whether or not they are useful in practice.

Every healthcare professional should participate in some form of research. Forms of participation include:

- contributing to an idea for a clinical study by identifying a situation in need of change or a problem that exists in practice
- acting as a member of a research team, whether assisting in obtaining consent from participants or collecting data
- advising colleagues, patients or clients about participating in research
- seeking answers to problems in your work environment, be it clinical or otherwise, by searching for or appraising existing research evidence
- undertaking an independent research project
- being an active user of research findings
- engaging in discussions of research findings by participating in a journal club
- acting as an advocate for patients (where patients are involved).

Using research knowledge to promote evidence-based practice

Health sciences research has developed significantly over the last 50 years. Greater emphasis is placed on the assimilation and application of research findings in practice in order to promote quality outcomes for patients, the community, healthcare providers and the healthcare system as a whole.

Leaders in the field accept the value of research and EBP, but are concerned about the extent to which healthcare professionals utilise and draw upon research findings to guide decisions about patient care. In the past, healthcare practices and management protocols were seldom questioned by those outside the field. However, consumers and patients have become more assertive and have added their voices to the demand that clinical practice be based on scientific evidence. This is also the case for educational and managerial practices in the healthcare environment.

It is essential that research be put into practice: health sciences researchers must ensure that professionals understand and use the evidence they make available. Putting research into practice entails much more than merely conducting research projects in practice – it is about doing the right research and ensuring that the findings are valued and implemented (Clifford & Clark, 2004; Harvey & Land, 2021).

During the mid-90s, in the United Kingdom (UK), the National Health Service (NHS) Executive Report (1996) proposed three main functions in the achievement of clinical efficacy in practice: inform, change and monitor. It is important that healthcare professionals remain aware of the importance of clinical efficacy, and they should be encouraged to use this information to review their practices. They must monitor and assess the effects of change to ensure improvements in the quality-of-care result. In the past the dissemination of published research was fairly limited. The last three decades, however, have seen research results being increasingly incorporated in practice. Furthermore, researchers, committed decision-makers, research funders and educational institutions are more willing to consider collaboration to improve their practices.

Several factors have restricted health sciences research, including:
- Some healthcare professionals believe that they already carry out best practice. If a particular method has not been problematic, they continue to use it.
- Some healthcare professionals have alienated themselves from research. This may be due to negative experiences, lack of knowledge or a lack of interest in improving practice on a continuous basis.
- Lack of a research culture in a particular environment. A research-based culture continues to be a rarity for some healthcare professionals.
- The quantitative research versus qualitative research debate has hindered the field.
- Healthcare professionals are often used by other researchers as data collectors only.

Definition of evidence-based practice

All healthcare professionals have a moral and ethical obligation to ensure that the care they render is based on the best available evidence and is of the highest quality possible. EBP aims to deliver efficient and appropriate care to every patient or client. Sackett, Strauss, Richardson, Rosenberg and Haynes (2000: 1) posit that evidence-based medicine (EBM) 'is the integration of best research evidence with clinical expertise and patient values'. Harvey and Land (2021) describe EBP as a 'structured and objective approach to determine the best evidence upon which care should be based'. EBP has four elements: the best research evidence at the time, the values and preferences of the patient or client, the knowledge and expertise of the healthcare professional, and the best resources available.

Evidence forms the core of EBP. Healthcare professionals work with many types of evidence, of which research constitutes the strongest. Since research aims to answer specific research questions, the answers may not be relevant in all cases or settings. It is therefore important that the healthcare professional carefully consider the context, clinical setting, resources and patient preferences, together with the evidence, when making a decision about individual patient care (Newhouse et al, 2007).

The evidence-based decision-making process enables healthcare professionals to ensure they remain up to date in their clinical expertise. 'Clinical expertise' implies the ability of a healthcare professional to use their clinical skills and experience to identify a patient's health problems and needs, the patient's values and expectations, and the benefit of potential interventions in order to treat the patient as well as possible. To assist in the decision-making process the following questions could be asked:

- Is the outcome satisfactory and the best we can achieve?
- What is my judgement about the nature of the problem and how it can be addressed?
- What would be the best intervention in this particular instance?
- Which treatments are worth the cost when using them?
- How good is the evidence for using this particular intervention or treatment?

These questions could be rephrased to suit a particular problem or situation. For example, a health sciences educator may ask these questions related to assessment practices for first-year students. Or a health services manager may ask the questions to suit a human resources problem that may be experienced in a hospital.

Healthcare professionals should use a combination of clinical expertise and the most recent and relevant research – neither is adequate on its own. Without clinical expertise, practice risks being usurped by evidence. Without current research-based evidence, practice risks becoming outdated. Both these factors are detrimental to patient care (Grove, Gray & Burns, 2018).

The hierarchy of evidence

It is often difficult to decide what good evidence is, and whether it is sound or reliable. Evidence can originate from a variety of sources, such as one's personal experience, the experience of others or systematic research. Each of these is valuable, but also has limitations. A healthcare professional's personal experience is sometimes the only evidence available. Validating the quality of one's experience is difficult because it is influenced by personal values and norms. In cases where no validated evidence is available healthcare professionals should trust their experience and use it for the patient's benefit.

Using 'expert' knowledge assumes that some individuals, because of their cumulative experience and clinical expertise, have extensive knowledge or skills in a particular sphere. There are, of course, problems with this type of evidence. First, unless there are ways to confirm the validity and reliability of the evidence, it could prove fallible in some instances. Secondly, 'expert' status is a socially constructed perception, and may be incorrect. Thirdly, perceived expertise makes for authority that may be difficult to challenge. For example, for a long time it has been the expert opinion of obstetricians that elective episiotomy is preferable to spontaneous perineal tearing. This 'expert opinion' has been disseminated through textbooks and has been built into routine practice and education. Evidence has since changed this opinion.

Investigative questions, gathering and analysing data, and validating findings all contribute to research-based evidence. These skills require critical thinking. Although both quantitative and qualitative research must convince the readers that the study effectively answers the questions, and that the results can be believed, the decisions at each stage of the research are selected by individuals whose world view and values have been shaped within a particular social and professional context. The applicability of results in wider spheres may be affected by, among others, a small sample size or contextual factors. Particular problems are encountered when a number of studies addressing an issue present conflicting results.

EBP is a process of lifelong, self-directed learning in which patient care is central. It creates a need for information about diagnosis, prognosis, therapy and other clinical and healthcare issues. During this process, healthcare professionals engage in the following:

- converting information needs into answerable questions
- locating adequate evidence with which to answer research questions, by means of clinical examination, diagnostics or published literature
- critically appraising evidence for validity, usefulness or clinical applicability
- critically appraising evidence for practices related to the education and training of healthcare professionals and managing health facilities as these services directly affect quality of care
- integrating results of appraisals with clinical expertise and applying them to clinical practice
- evaluating clinical performance.

In order to determine the importance of evidence a hierarchy of evidence has been proposed. The hierarchical system provides a relative weight/importance to the evidence which is based on the particular study design and methodology used. Generally, the higher on the hierarchy a methodology is ranked, the more vigorous it is assumed to be. Meta-analysis, by synthesising the results of several similar clinical trials to produce a result of higher statistical power, is regarded as the highest level of evidence. The bottom level of evidence is obtained from individual case reports, regarded as providing the weakest level of evidence. The levels of hierarchy are from top to bottom: (1) systematic reviews, (2) randomised controlled trials, (3) cohort studies and case series studies, (4) qualitative studies, and (5) opinions.

This hierarchical structure should, however, not be seen as the only way to rank evidence. The topic, context and purpose of the study and its outcomes often determine the relevance to practice. Techniques lower down the ranking are not always redundant or unnecessary. Harvey and Land (2021) provide a classic example of research that was conducted through a lower-ranked process, but is still regarded as important. They refer to the study on the link between smoking and lung cancer that was initially discovered via case-control studies carried out in the 1950s. Although randomised controlled trials (RCTs) are considered more robust, it would have been unethical to perform an RCT. For example, if studying a risk factor exposure, you would need a cohort exposed to the risk factor by chance or personal choice.

The ranking system is also not unqualified and focuses mostly on quantitative methodologies. A poorly conducted RCT on specific treatment plans will provide less compelling evidence than a well-conducted observational study. It is important that the most appropriate study design is used to answer the question.

Systematic, integrative and scoping reviews

Evidence can be integrated in many ways, with the literature review being a well-known option. However, the focus has shifted towards a more systematic and critical way of summarising evidence. A systematic review entails a scientific, comprehensive synthesis of quantitative and outcome-based studies in particular healthcare disciplines to determine the best research evidence available (Grove, Gray & Burns, 2018; Polit & Beck, 2021). A unique feature of a systematic review is the critical appraisal of the methodological quality of studies found applicable to the review question.

High-quality reviews take great care to find all relevant studies, published and unpublished, to assess each study's methodological quality, to synthesise the findings from individual studies in an unbiased way and to present a balanced and impartial summary of the findings with due consideration of any flaws in the evidence (Harvey & Land, 2021; How & Crombie, 2001). A review can only be as good as the studies included therein. In the case of poor-quality reviews, the findings may be misleading. You should read any systematic and/or integrative review with a critical mind and remain sceptical.

Various types of reviews can be done. These are the three most used reviews:

- A systematic review is an exact synthesis of all investigations related to one specific question, focusing primarily on experimental studies, such as RCTs, aiming at overcoming possible biases in each stage, following a strict method to search and select investigations; assessing relevance and validity of the studies found; collection, synthesis and interpretation of data from research.
- An integrative review proposes to integrate the literature found on a determined object of investigation and is the most comprehensive methodological approach of reviews.
- Scoping reviews aim to map the literature, seeking to describe the results in a graphic and classificatory way to have a better idea on what information is available on a particular topic.

One may feel that it is impossible or difficult to find the appropriate evidence. However, the hierarchical guidelines are constructed in such a way that one should engage in a thorough investigation of all the evidence on a particular topic. It is important to understand how rigorously one should consider evidence before adopting or rejecting it.

Summary

This chapter was an introduction to health sciences research. The meaning of research and the main types of research were presented from various points of view, and the differences between the major features of quantitative and qualitative research were explained. Reasons for conducting research and the roles of healthcare professionals in research were discussed. Lastly, a brief exploration of evidence-based practice was outlined.

Exercises

1. Think back about all the instances where you were part of research. Group the activities or experiences according to what your role was. For example, were you part of an opinion poll, were you a participant in a focus group or were you part of the data collection team? What have you learned from this experience?

2. Write down a definition of research in your own words. Then compare it to the conceptual definition of research.

3. Consider one or two facts that you know and trace these back to their source. Is the basis of your knowledge tradition, authority, logical reasoning, experience or scientific research? Justify your answer.

4. Discuss barriers to the implementation of research in your workplace.

5. You wish to study the health perceptions of women in underprivileged, poverty-stricken areas. Would this topic lend itself best to a qualitative or a quantitative research study? Provide a rationale.

6. Find at least one article that used each of the methodologies according to the hierarchical structure. Read the articles and reflect on the value of the evidence for you in your particular work environment. Indicate how you would rank the articles based on their appropriateness for you.

7. Search, find and read at least two systematic and/or integrative reviews and debate the value thereof with a colleague.

Research and theory

Chapter 2

LEARNING OUTCOMES

On completion of this chapter, you should be able to demonstrate your understanding of:

- theory, paradigm, metaparadigm, philosophy, model, framework, concept, construct and proposition
- four types of theory
- the differences between theoretical and conceptual frameworks
- the steps used in theory development
- the steps used in theory testing
- the relationship between research and theory

Theories are systematic explanations of aspects of reality. Theories integrate concepts into a coherent system in research. This chapter focuses on **scientific theory**. Scientific theory has extensive evidence of valid and reliable methods for measuring each concept and the relational statements. From these relationships, propositions can be developed and tested. The relationship between research and theory, as well as the relationship between research and practice, is based on interdependence and inseparability. Research is guided by theory and depends on its ability to increase understanding. In turn, theory relies on carefully conducted research to give its concepts and frameworks credibility. It is, however, also true that scientific theories remain open to possible opposing evidence that would require careful consideration.

The nature of scientific theory

In scientific research, theories are systematically and rigorously formulated and tested. They reflect current understandings of phenomena and may change as new knowledge is discovered and updated. A recent example of a theory being reconsidered is the change in the knowledge pertaining to functions and interactions of various genes. Extensive research on the human genomes has yielded new information about genetics and how to treat diseases. Another example centres around the concept of ageing: the 'disengagement theory' asserts that people deliberately withdraw from all types of social interactions as they grow older, while the 'activity theory' challenges this notion by proposing that older people want to remain active in all aspects of their lives. The theory also suggests that any withdrawal is involuntary. Recent research supports the activity theory. Researchers belonging to the Association of Internet Researchers and who hold deontological perspectives to research support the Kantian deontological theory that gives priority to adapting, updating and clarifying codes to make sure researchers use appropriate guidelines for ethical conduct. These researchers follow guidelines as closely as possible when doing online research, even if it means following the rules that were created for conventional research and adjusting online research rules (Salmons, 2016).

Definitions of theory

Theories are used to organise a body of knowledge and to establish what is known about a phenomenon. There are many definitions of 'theory' in the health sciences. Some are narrow and specific, while others are broad and generic. Moreover, several concepts used interchangeably describe the same concept. They include: 'conceptual framework', 'conceptual model', 'paradigm', 'metaparadigm', 'theoretical framework' and 'theoretical perspective'. However, not all of these terms are equally accurate or descriptive. Polit and Beck (2021) argue that while a conceptual model is similar to a theory, it is also more abstract. It is thus imperative for researchers to clarify the context in which a selected term is used.

Gray (2021) states that a theory consists of a set of interrelated concepts, definitions and propositions that demonstrate relationships between variables. Chinn and Kramer describe theory as a 'systematic abstraction of reality that serves some purpose' (Chinn & Kramer, 2011). 'Systematic' implies a specific organisational pattern, 'abstraction' refers to a representation of reality and 'purposes' include description, explanation and prediction of phenomena, as well as control of reality. A theory thus summarises and organises understanding of a particular phenomenon and can be systematically tested by research. It presents a systematic explanation about the relationships among phenomena (Polit & Beck, 2021). Examples with which you may already be familiar include Maslow's hierarchy of needs, Rosenstock's health belief model and Selye's theory of physiological adaptation to stress.

Types of theory

There are several types of theory, including metatheory, grand theory, factor-isolating theory, descriptive theory and practice theory. Theories are classified primarily according to their purpose or scope, or according to their breadth or level of abstraction. Several authors use the latter classification and depict the scope or level of abstraction according to hierarchical levels from broad to limited, as shown in Figure 2.1 (Burns & Grove, 2019; Chinn & Kramer, 2015; Moody, 1990; Walker & Avant, 2015; Wilson, 2014).

The highest level depicted in Figure 2.1 is metatheory, which refers to both theorising about theory as well as the process of theory development. Its focus is broad and includes a variety of analyses of the purposes and types of theory required for research at the highest levels. An example of a metatheory would be that 'caring' is a key concept in nursing, and that 'nursing' is the study of caring in the human health experience, where the environment is inherent in, and inseparable from, the integrated focus of caring.

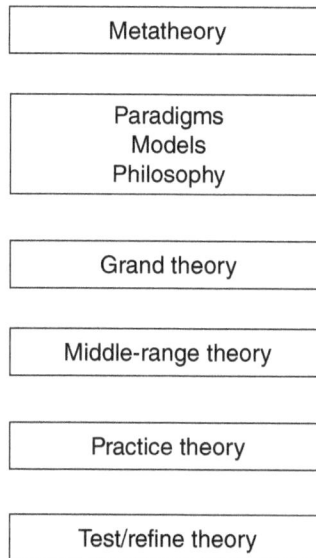

Metatheory

Paradigms
Models
Philosophy

Grand theory

Middle-range theory

Practice theory

Test/refine theory

Figure 2.1 Levels of theory

Grand theories provide a global perspective about a discipline and its scope of practice. As a rule, these theories are so abstract that they do not lend themselves to direct empirical testing. Some writers consider them synonymous with conceptual models and paradigms (Burns & Grove, 2020; Moody, 1990; Polit & Beck, 2021; Stevens-Barnum, 1990). To Merton (1968), a sociologist who first proposed grand and middle-range theories, the former are the core of a science and are not testable because they represent conceptual frameworks. To build grand theories a body of knowledge related to a particular theory is required and involves both an organised research programme and a team of researchers.

Middle-range theories are generally more focused in scope than grand theories. They deal with circumscribed phenomena, such as pain, stress, coping mechanisms and chemical dependence, within a clearly defined context. Propositions are clearly formulated, and testable hypotheses can be derived. Middle-range theory is generally more practical, applicable and easier to test, confirm or refute in empirical research than grand theory. It is one of the most useful theories in health sciences research.

The distinguishing features of grand and middle-range theories are evident in this example. Looking at a theory of health or high-level wellness, you would probably note that it represents ideas that have been put together in a unique way to describe or explain health or high-level wellness. Such a theory is evidently useful for the health sciences because it facilitates an understanding of the world in terms of one of the health sciences' major concerns, that is, health. Moreover, it frames the way in which we can view health or high-level wellness and suggests the direction that a research project dealing with related concepts should take. The theory provides a global perspective of health; in other words, it considers all of the health sciences' concerns with health and high-level wellness. Therefore, it applies to individuals in general and not to a particular individual in a specific situation. Health and high-level wellness are abstract concepts and can have various definitions. Thus, the theory that pertains to these concepts is regarded as a 'grand theory'.

By contrast, a theory of pain alleviation or stress management deals with only one part of health sciences' concern with health and high-level wellness. In this theory a definitive piece of reality is suggested in a concrete manner, which is much less vague than the information provided by a grand theory. A clearer theory is easily tested, confirmed or refuted in the empirical world, and may therefore be called a middle-range theory.

A theory that deals with one person in a particular situation at a certain point in time is described as **narrow-range** or **micro-theory**. Concepts contained in this type of theory are intensely focused, specifically defined and applicable only to certain instances or test cases. An example of such a theory could be the interactions between individuals, such as the relationship between adult children and their parents.

Practice theory is characterised by its goal of prescriptive action. The classic division proposed by Dickhoff and James (1968: 202) identifies four levels of practice theory. The lower levels are developed first and provide a basis for the higher ones. The levels in ascending order are:

1. *Factor-isolating theory*, which focuses on observing, describing and naming concepts. This leads the researcher to construct the factor-isolating or concept-naming theory. This level is also known as the 'descriptive level'.
2. *Factor-relating theory*, which takes the isolated concepts a step further and relates them to one another. Description is still the purpose of the study, but at this level it focuses on the relationships between the concepts.
3. *Situation-relating theory*, which explains the relationships between the concepts or propositions. The researcher attempts to answer the question, 'What will happen if …?' and accordingly designs a study to test the relationships.
4. *Situation-producing theory*, which requires the specification of an activity as well as its goal. This theory is also referred to as a 'prescriptive theory', as it prescribes what the healthcare professional must do to attain a desired goal. The question here is: 'How can I make this happen?' Thus the purpose of this level of theory is predictive.

Theory-related terms

The concepts of metaparadigm, paradigm, models, frameworks and philosophy are increasingly prevalent in literature dealing with health sciences research.

Paradigm

Paradigms for human inquiry refer to ways in which people respond to basic philosophical questions. Laudan (1995) and Polit and Beck (2021) describe a paradigm as a worldview and a set of assumptions about the basic kinds of entities in the world, how these entities interact, and the proper methods to use for constructing and testing theories of these entities. So, paradigms are characterised in terms of their specific ontological, epistemological and methodological assumptions (Polit & Beck, 2021).

The assumptions that describe a specific paradigm were described by Guba (1990) as:

- **Ontology** – a patterned set of assumptions about reality. It consists of a set of concepts and categories in a subject area or domain that show their properties and the relations between them. Ontology therefore seeks the classification and explanation of entities.
- **Epistemology** – knowledge of that reality. It is described as the theory of knowledge, especially about its scope, methods and validity, and the distinction between justified belief and opinion. Epistemology therefore is the philosophical study of the nature, origin and limits of human knowledge.
- **Methodology** – the particular ways of knowing about that reality. Methodology entails an outline of how a given study is carried out. It denotes the techniques or procedures that are used to identify and analyse information regarding a specific research topic.

Polit and Beck (2021: 9) state that 'paradigms for human inquiry are often characterised in terms of the ways in which they respond to basic philosophical questions, such as:

- **Ontologic:** What is the nature of reality?
- **Epistemologic:** What is the relationship between the inquirer and [the phenomenon] being studied?
- **Methodologic:** How should the inquirer obtain knowledge?'

These assumptions are untested 'givens' that guide and influence the researcher's investigation. They must decide what assumptions are acceptable and appropriate and must use methods consistent with a specific paradigm to guide them. The three main paradigmatic approaches relevant to science are 'positivism', 'critical theory' and 'interpretivism'. **Positivism** is a systematic research method which emphasises the importance of observable facts. **Critical theory** is an approach to social science which emphasises the need to uncover 'hidden' processes and structures within society. For example, critical theorists reject the notion that actions be taken for granted. These theorists would provide various interpretations to 'silence' in that it could be the absence of a response, absence of communication between people or speaking quietly. **Interpretivism** is another social science approach. It emphasises the importance of insiders' viewpoints in understanding social environments and phenomena. It focuses on the meaning that individuals or communities assign to their experiences.

Paradigms are about worldviews, methodological ideals, social communities or academic societies (Alvesson & Sandberg, 2021). According to Moody (1990), a prominent health sciences researcher of the 1990s, paradigms assist the researcher to be organised in their thinking, observing and interpreting processes. In essence, a paradigm frames the way in which a discipline's concerns are viewed and the direction a research project takes. A paradigm structures the questions which need to be posed, eliminates questions that are external to its conceptual boundaries, provides a link to specific research methods, and suggests criteria with which the researcher can assess the appropriateness of research tools.

A paradigm is a means to examine natural phenomena. It encompasses a set of philosophical assumptions which guide the researcher's approach to inquiry (Polit & Beck, 2021). A paradigm is thus an over-arching philosophical framework which supports the production of scientific knowledge. A paradigm serves as a 'lens' or organised principles through which a researcher approaches and interprets reality. However, several authors caution that there are also disadvantages to accepting a dominant paradigm (Feyerabend, 1975; Moody, 1990; Wilson, 1989). Feyerabend (1975) provides two reasons: first, epistemological prescriptions do not guarantee the best way of discovering isolated facts. Secondly, where education follows a rigid scientific process, the humanity could get lost as it is not suitable and adaptable to the uniqueness of the individuals or groups involved. Moody (1990) and Wilson (1989) also oppose an unquestioning adherence to a particular paradigm, as they believe that this may blind us to discoveries, delay scientific progress, and make us prisoners of our own paradigms. Thus, healthcare practice demands multiple paradigms for interpreting observations and providing structure to systematic study. More recently, authors have written widely about the paradigm or paradigms used in mixed-methods research that is characterised by meta-inferences in that conclusions are drawn from both qualitative and quantitative discoveries (Bergman, 2010; Creamer, 2018; Creswell & Creswell, 2018; Creswell & Plano Clark, 2018; Polit & Beck, 2021). Bergman (2010) explains that scientific paradigms determine the type of questions researchers pose, how these questions are to be addressed, what data is collected, and how the findings are interpreted to derive answers to these questions. In research, where one is faced with two different paradigms, such as in mixed-methods research, one would consider a new or different paradigm, not merely two competing paradigms. Rather, these researchers seek distinctions in the construction of meaning of concepts in relation to how participants understand or make sense of their experiences or report on their views in questionnaires, respectively.

Multiple paradigms exist and authors group them differently and provide different views of what the main paradigms are.

Polit and Beck (2021: 7) explain paradigms by posing the following questions: 'What is the nature of reality?' and 'What is the relationship between the inquirer and those being studies?' These authors group paradigms as follows:

- Positivist paradigm (including postpositivist paradigm).
- Constructivist paradigm (also called naturalist paradigm). Naturalism is an extension of the transformation called postmodernism. Postmodern thinking has emphasised the value of deconstructing old ideas and structures and reconstructing ideas and structures into new ways of thinking and doing.
- Transformative paradigm that underpins critical theory research.
- Pragmatist paradigm that underpins mixed methods research.

Leavy (2017) groups paradigms as

- postpositivist paradigm
- interpretive/constructivist paradigm
- critical paradigm
- transformative paradigm
- pragmatic paradigm
- arts-based/aesthetic intersubjective paradigm.

Du Plooy-Cilliers et al (2014: 23) explain three dominant research traditions as being:

- positivism – the cognitive interest of this paradigm lies in empirical-analytical sciences. The aim is to find causal relationships (cause and effect).
- interpretivism – the cognitive interest of this paradigm lies in the historical-hermeneutic or hermeneutic-phenomenological sciences. The interest lies in an in-depth understanding of a phenomenon and practical sciences. This type of science is related to interpretivism.
- critical realism – the cognitive interest lies in emancipatory realism. The aim is to empower people through knowledge.

It is important for researchers to determine their theoretical position in terms of the phenomenon under investigation. The question is also about the techniques that researchers will use to structure their study. The research question will guide how data will be gathered and analysed. Only then can the researcher determine how to view the complexity of the phenomenon. The selected paradigm for an inquiry is characterised in terms of the way in which a researcher will respond to questions about the nature of reality and the relationships between the researcher and the researched.

Metaparadigm

The paradigm is a vital concept steering the development of a scientific discipline. Paradigms that shape the education, research and practice steps of a discipline (such as health sciences) are defined as metaparadigms. The term 'metaparadigm' is derived from Kuhn's (1970) original work on paradigms. The metaparadigm constitutes a discipline's global perspective and serves as an encapsulating framework within which more defined models, paradigms or theories develop. Each discipline's metaparadigm specifies its distinct perspective. The general consensus among health sciences scholars is that the concepts of person, health, environment and action comprise the major health sciences' metaparadigms (Deliktas et al, 2019; Moody, 1990; Newman, 1983; Wilson, 1989; Yura & Torres, 1975; Polit & Beck, 2021). In relation to nursing, Watson (2008; 2021) considers nursing care to be the core indicator of nursing practice and suggests nursing care as the fifth metaparadigm. Metaparadigms, or dominant paradigms, therefore, are regarded as general parameters of a scientific discipline and focus on scientific efforts. Metaparadigms may include several concrete and specific paradigms for researchers.

Philosophy

The term 'philosophy' refers to 'worldview' and is described as rational intellectual explorations of truths, or principles of being, knowledge or conduct (Grove et al, 2015). It denotes our assumptions, values and beliefs about the nature of reality, knowledge and methods of obtaining knowledge. Philosophical underpinning of research is one of the three elements of research (philosophical, praxis and ethics). The philosophical underpinning entails three foundations: paradigm, ontology and epistemology. The philosophical elements of research address the question: 'What do we believe?' At the level of praxis lies design, methods and theory. The ethical component includes the philosophical and praxis elements, and includes values, ethical considerations and reflexivity (Leavy, 2017).

Model

This term is used somewhat inconsistently in health sciences literature. While it is sometimes used interchangeably with 'theory', some writers distinguish between the two and view a model as a **precursor** of a theory (Mouton, 1996). Polit and Beck (2021) use the terms 'model', 'conceptual frameworks' and 'conceptual schemes' interchangeably.

A model is defined as a symbolic depiction of reality. It provides a schematic representation of relationships among phenomena and uses symbols or diagrams to represent an idea. Concepts are assembled by virtue of their relevance to a common theme. Models help us structure the way we view situations, events or groups of people. In health sciences research, models may help to define and guide specific research tasks or provide organised frameworks. Models are not formally tested like theories, but provide perspective regarding interrelated phenomena and the dynamics of the relationships between concepts. Models provide a basic illustration of a process that could assist in understanding the nature of theories, constructs and concepts in a particular context. The visual depiction of concepts and their relationships illustrate the 'what' and 'how' of complex concepts (Du Plooy-Cilliers et al, 2014: 48). Models, however, lack the 'why' of the concepts, which is explained in a theory.

Frameworks

A framework is an abstract, logical structure of meaning, guiding the development of the study and enabling the researcher to link the findings to a particular body of knowledge. A research study's framework helps to organise the study and provides a context in which the researcher examines a problem and gathers and analyses data. A distinction is frequently made between theoretical and conceptual frameworks (Gray, Grove & Sutherland, 2017; Grey, 2021; Nieswiadomy, 2012; Polit & Beck, 2021). A **theoretical framework** is based on propositional statements resulting from an existing theory and integrates observations and facts into an orderly scheme, while a conceptual framework is developed through identifying and defining concepts and proposing relationships between them. Both frameworks connect concepts to create a specific way of looking at a phenomenon. By developing a framework within which ideas are organised, the researcher can demonstrate that the proposed study is a logical extension of current knowledge.

Not all studies are based on formal theories or conceptual models. Every study, however, has a framework providing conceptual rationale. Frameworks may be implicit without being formally described. This may result in inadequate explanations of concepts and relationships between concepts. Frameworks could be derived from the literature by conducting a thorough literature review on the topic of interest or a well-tested theory. It is important that the 'fit' between the study variables and the selected framework is as snug as possible. The framework should apply to every step of the research process.

Many theories are used as frameworks. For example, a healthcare professional is concerned about incontinence in anxious children and wants to plan a study to modify this. She selects a behavioural theory – Skinner's reinforcement theory – for the purposes of her research. She posits that incontinence is a behaviour characterised by involuntary urination before a patient can get to a toilet or be positioned on a bedpan. Skinner's theory suggests that behaviour can be modified through reinforcement. The healthcare professional thus hypothesises that patients can be taught to control urination if effective reinforcers, such as appropriate rewards, are applied.

Other theories frequently used as frameworks are Rosenstock's health belief model, Pender's health promotion model and Selye's stress theory, as well as the nursing theories of authorities such as Orem, King, Neumann, Leininger, and so on.

Once a researcher has identified a suitable conceptual framework, they should evaluate its usefulness by answering the following questions:
- Is the theory/framework appropriate to the research problem?
- Is the theory/framework congruent to your beliefs and values?

In purely qualitative studies the research problem may not be explained in terms of theoretical or conceptual frameworks. The researcher may instead employ a philosophical rationale or central theoretical statement to examine the problem.

Development of theory

A researcher's first step in developing a theory is for them to become familiar with its structural and functional components. The **structural components** include assumptions, concepts, constructs, variables and propositions. The **functional components** consist of the domain concepts of the theory and how you should use them, that is, describe, explain, predict or control in order to operationalise the concepts.

Assumptions are principles that we accept to be true without proof or verification and are taken for granted. They are often entrenched in thinking and behaviour. They determine our understanding of concepts, definitions, purposes and relationships. Assumptions form the basis from which theoretical reasoning proceeds. In research, assumptions are embedded in the philosophical bases of framework, design and the interpretation of findings, and influence a study's logic (Grey, 2021; Grove et al, 2013).

Concepts are linguistic labels we assign to objects or events. They can be described as the 'building blocks' of theories and as 'abstractions of particular aspects of human behaviour and characteristics' (Polit & Beck, 2021). Concepts vary in levels of abstraction. Examples of highly abstract, complex concepts include those of 'self-esteem' and 'coping' – both of which are difficult to measure. Less abstract concepts, such as weight gain or weight loss, and blood loss, lend themselves to empirical measurements. Generally, the more abstract and complex the concept is, the more difficult it is for the researcher to derive valid and reliable empirical data.

Concepts are not always clearly defined or clarified in general usage. For example, when a patient describes themselves as 'sad' and you know what is making them feel that way, the description may be sufficient for you to understand what the patient means. However, if you were to study the concept of 'sadness' in more detail, you would have to define, specify and clarify the emotion. Defining concepts properly ensures that terms are used consistently.

When a concept is clarified (so that it is potentially observable) and in a form that is measurable, it is considered a **construct**. For example, a construct associated with the concept of 'pain' may be physiological and psychological discomfort. Constructs are deliberately non-specific, and healthcare professionals who deal with them understand what to measure, observe or control.

Variables are more precise and specific than both concepts and constructs. They imply that a concept can be accurately defined so that precise observations and measurements are possible. Figure 2.2 shows how a proposition can be developed.

Propositions, sometimes referred to as 'relational statements', suggest a specific relationship between or among two or more concepts or constructs. The nature of the relationship can take various forms. Concepts can be related to others, or they can be completely unrelated. General propositions could include where emotional stress is associated with psychological responses to the environment. A more specific proposition would be where emotional stress is associated with blood pressure. Concepts may also be related negatively or positively. For example, a relationship specifically indicating that since it shows the 'connection' between these concepts, emotional stress increases blood pressure, would be regarded as a positive relationship.

Proposition: as pain increases, muscle tension increases

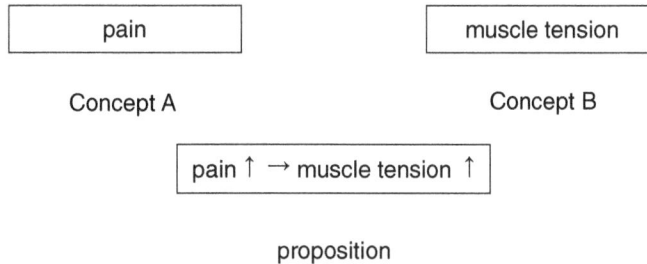

pain		muscle tension
Concept A		Concept B

pain ↑ → muscle tension ↑

proposition

Figure 2.2 Proposition development

Propositions provide the substance and form of a theory. Figure 2.3 illustrates the links between concepts, constructs and variables.

	Example 1	Example 2	Levels of abstraction
Concept	pain	anxiety	abstract
Construct	physiological and psychological discomfort resulting from internal or external stressors	emotional response	abstract
Variable	the score obtained on the pain inventory self-test	palmar sweating	concrete

Figure 2.3 The links between concepts, constructs and variables

Theory development requires a systematic process of inquiry. Chinn and Kramer (2015) outline several steps to the process:

1. Identify, select and clarify concepts.
2. Identify assumptions which form the basis of the theory.
3. Clarify the context.
4. Develop relational statements through concept analysis, derivation or synthesis.
5. Test relational statements and validate relationships.

These steps need not be performed in any specific order. In practice, however, there is a flow of thought from one step to another as ideas are developed and refined.

There are numerous approaches to developing theory, most of which are shaped by logical positivist views where one wants to understand the underlying causes of phenomena. Imagination and creativity are desirable in all approaches to theory building. Examples of those used in the health sciences include: induction, deduction and retroduction, theory derivation, model confirmation, and borrowing and building with metaphors.

Testing of theory

Any health sciences theory should be useful for the practice. Because theories are abstractions of reality, they must be tested to ensure that they represent the real world. The process of testing theory involves defining concepts so that they can be measured, that is, developing operational definitions of concepts and then devising propositions and hypotheses. These hypotheses are predictions about how variables would be related if the theory were correct. A theory is never tested directly, but the hypotheses deduced from the theory are subjected to scientific investigation.

The major focus of the testing process is the comparison of observed research outcomes and relationships predicted by the hypotheses. The theory is thus continually subjected to potential disconfirmation through this process. The repeated failure of research endeavours to disconfirm a theory results in increased support for, and acceptance of, the theory.

The relationship between theory and research

Health sciences research and theory are interdependent and inseparable. Theory is a generalised concept which provides an explanation of existing 'things', while research is a way of expanding the existing knowledge base and creating new knowledge. Research validates and modifies theory. Theories could be used to formulate a set of generalisations to explain relationships among variables. When empirically tested, the results of the research can be used to verify, modify, disprove or support a theoretical proposition. Theory guides and generates research ideas, while research assesses the value of existing theory and provides a foundation on which new theory is built. Theories allow researchers to combine observations and facts into an orderly system. They guide the researcher's understanding of phenomena as well as the reasons behind their occurrence. Theories therefore help to stimulate research and extend knowledge by providing both direction and impetus.

Research plays an active role in theory development. It initiates, reformulates, deflects and clarifies theory. Theory and research are thus mutually beneficial. Moody (1990) describes the theory–research relationship as 'concatenated'. This means that they are both linked within each series of events in the theory–research process. Indeed, Stevens-Barnum (1990) and Polit and Beck (2021) posit that research and theory are interrelated and form a cyclic chain in which theory directs research, research corrects theory, and corrected (or confirmed) theory directs further research.

However, the interrelatedness of theory and research is not always evident in health sciences research. Healthcare professionals have been, and continue to be, criticised for producing numerous instances of isolated research results which are difficult to integrate into existing bodies of knowledge owing to the absence of a theoretical foundation. Although this may hinder the development of the field, it would be unreasonable to assert that research without theoretical underpinning cannot make a contribution to science. In some cases, research findings may be so pragmatic that they do not need a theory to enhance their usefulness. Indeed, non-theoretical research can potentially be linked to theory at a later stage.

Summary

In this chapter we focused on the relationship between theory and research, referring to the various meanings attributed to theory and related terms in the health sciences research literature. Having provided and compared several definitions of the term 'theory', we then outlined the different theories themselves, as described in the literature, and explored the definitions of terms related to theory. We paid attention to theory development and testing, and briefly discussed the steps used in both. Finally, we confirmed the interdependent nature of the relationship between theory and research.

Exercises

1. Draw a table differentiating between the different paradigms. Think of an example of a research question that will best suit each paradigm.

2. Search for three existing theories and give an example of a study that you would plan, using each of these theories. You could use articles to serve as an example, but devise your own example of a study that you could embark on, using that particular theory.

3. Select a research article which describes a study guided by a conceptual or theoretical framework. Analyse how the framework influenced the research process.

4. How would you convince a fellow researcher to use a framework, whether theoretical or conceptual?

5. Critically read your selected research article and describe the theoretical frameworks that the researcher used.

Ethical considerations in the conduct of health sciences research

LEARNING OUTCOMES

On completion of this chapter, you should be able to demonstrate your understanding of:

- the basic ethics of delivering healthcare
- the basic ethical principles underlying protection of human participants
- legislation related to research
- the rights of human participants that need to be recognised and protected by the researcher
- the essential elements of an informed consent form, which complies with principles of research ethics and protects the rights of human participants
- the adequacy of a consent form
- the factors that affect human participants who are particularly vulnerable to risk in research
- appropriate steps that the researcher must take in working with vulnerable groups
- the risks and benefits associated with research procedures
- steps that the researcher should take to safeguard the anonymity and confidentiality of research participants
- the role of institutional review boards and committees in the review of research proposals and reports
- the ethical implications of a research report

A researcher must have the necessary tools to understand what ethics is about. Questions about how we should understand ethical problems or dilemmas and how we make ethical choices or decisions in research should be asked constantly. There are constant shifts in the social and health sciences contexts that require one to reconsider, rethink and re-debate what constitutes ethical practice. Changes such as an increase in online research as well as healthcare changes resulting from the Covid-19 pandemic and the move to assisted dying force us to ask questions continuously.

A researcher must understand the importance of protecting research participants. The benefit of the research must outweigh its risk. The concept of the risk–benefit ratio will be discussed in more detail later in this chapter. Researchers are accountable for their findings and are expected to promote the social and ethical values of all involved.

Researchers involved in research with human participants have special concerns related to the protection of human rights and to social well-being, particularly in lower- and middle-income and resource-constrained countries. It should also be remembered that our understanding of the ethical implications of research is originally based on Western values. However, researchers must engage in the decolonisation of research ethics especially related to consent. The current debate agrees that research involving indigenous people must be conducted with the collaboration, consultation and consent of the communities and community leaders. However, the implementation of this notion has practical challenges. Challenges include inherent methodological issues and indigenous governance of research. Of importance is that research institutions overseeing health research need to consider the indigenous practices affecting the communities that are involved in the research. Even though the research project has been approved by the institutional research ethics board and complies with the legal requirements, these communities still have the right to decline the request for research to be conducted in their communities. Researchers must seriously consider and respect the collective identity of indigenous communities and the research risk when planning research, and specifically do so in a co-constructed manner (Brunger et al, 2021).

Historically research ethics has been a continuous debate, involving the discovery of numerous research atrocities in the past. These atrocities prompted the development of stringent rules and regulations to protect participants. Should you want to read about these studies, you could search for the following: the Tuskegee Syphilis Study, the syphilis study in Guatemala, the Nazi experiments, and the thalidomide disaster (Moodley, 2017).

Research that lacks scientific or social value is unethical as it results in the exploitation of human participants by exposing them to potential harm and wastage of resources. Much work still has to be done for researchers to fully understand the impact of research and the meaning of autonomy, beneficence and privacy, for example. With the current debate on decolonisation in research and increased online research practices, researchers need to continuously question the practices and their relevance.

Codes of ethical research

The Nuremberg Code was the first set of guidelines aimed at protecting the rights of research participants. It mandated voluntary consent, justification of research for the good of society (with appropriate balance of risk and benefit), adequate protection of participants from risk or harm, the participant's right to withdraw from experimentation, and adequate scientific training for researchers (Moodley, 2017).

Although it was a good starting point, the code omitted two major classes of research participants: children and persons with mental disorders. The Declaration of Helsinki (first published in 1964 and amended most recently in 2013 by the World Medical Association) remedied this by incorporating conditions for the inclusion of children (only if parental permission is obtained) and persons who are mentally or intellectually challenged (if proxy consent is obtained). The Declaration distinguishes between therapeutic research, which benefits the research participant, and non-therapeutic research, which does not directly benefit the participant, and sets stringent constraints on researchers undertaking the latter. It also reiterates the Nuremberg Code and emphasises the importance of written consent.

Both the Nuremberg Code and the Declaration of Helsinki provide foundations for ethical research guidelines developed by governmental and professional organisations all over the world. The South African National Health Research Ethics Council (NHREC) was established in 2003 under the National Health Act 61 of 2003. The council provides direction on ethical issues related to health research and develops research guidelines.

While ethical principles relating to human participant protection play an important role in these documents, there are also other considerations. These include: honesty and integrity in conducting research, the researcher's responsibilities, sharing and utilising data, truthful reporting of results and conflicts of interest, as well as assigning authorship in scientific publications. Unethical research is rarely intentional, but can occur when participants' rights conflict with the demands of the research problems (Polit & Beck, 2021). For example, participants may experience serious adverse effects in the trial of a drug which could be a 'medical breakthrough'. Currently the debate around vaccination against the SARS-CoV-2 variants also raises ethical questions about potential adverse effects of being vaccinated, given the developments in these vaccines. The researcher thus needs to plan research around ethical principles and ensure that they adhere to them throughout the research process.

Fundamental ethical principles

Three fundamental ethical principles guide researchers: 'respect for persons/human dignity', 'beneficence' and 'justice'. These principles are based on human rights that need to be protected in research.

Principle of respect for persons/human dignity

Respect for human dignity includes the right to self-determination and the right to full disclosure. **Self-determination** refers to the right to decide voluntarily whether to participate in a study or not, without any risk of prejudice. Potential participants must be granted the right to ask questions, refuse to answer questions and withdraw from the study at any given time. Self-determination also means freedom from coercion. No implicit or explicit threats of penalty for failing to participate in a study or excessive rewards or remuneration for participating may occur. Coercion may also be subtle, especially where the researcher is in a position of authority in relation to the participant.

Another example of coercion may be where the participant is promised some form of remuneration, especially in poor communities where this could mean their only 'income' or a free meal. However, current practices in research allow for some form of incentive considered carefully to ensure that it is not coercion. Full disclosure refers to the right to make an informed decision to participate in a study after the researcher has fully described the study, the potential risks and benefits, and the right to refuse participation.

Full disclosure may result in biases and sample recruitment problems. For example, if a researcher wishes to study dishonesty in assessment, the students guilty of dishonesty might not agree to participate, once they know the research purpose. In this example, full disclosure of the research purpose could undermine the study. The researcher of this study could use concealment (covert data collection) where data is collected without the knowledge and consent of the participants (Polit & Beck, 2022). The data collection in this case could then, for example, be conducted through concealed methods such as observation while pretending to engage in other activities. Deception is a more controversial way of not fully disclosing the information about the study. It involves the deliberate withholding of information or providing participants with false information. Both concealment and deception are ethically problematic and interfere with the right to make a truly informed decision.

Current practices in researching data from the internet also pose questions for debate. For example, the question arises whether data from blogs or social media sites could be used without the consent of the authors. Some researchers argue that the blog is in the public domain once it is posted, whereas other researchers maintain that the same ethical principles apply in cyberspace research as bloggers are participants in online or virtual communities. The principle of doing no harm and the right to privacy should also be considered when making this decision.

This principle involves three convictions:
1. Individuals are autonomous: that is, they have the right to self-determination. Individuals can thus decide whether or not to participate in a study without the risk of penalty or prejudicial treatment. In addition, they have the right to withdraw at any time, to refuse to give information, and to ask for clarification about the purpose of the study. The researcher must respect these and avoid any form of coercion.
2. In some indigenous societies and religious groups, individuals may not be regarded as autonomous, and the researcher needs to respect traditional practices without disregarding the human rights of participants.
3. Individuals with diminished autonomy require additional protection. This group includes children, persons who are mentally or intellectually challenged, patients who are unconscious and patients who are institutionalised. In any scenario where power relations play a role the potential participant may be vulnerable to exploitation. The autonomy of children is described in various Acts and is country-specific.

Principle of beneficence

The principle of beneficence refers to the right to freedom from harm and discomfort and the right to protection from exploitation. To adhere to this principle the researcher needs to secure the participant's well-being. The participant has a right to be protected from discomfort and harm – whether physical, psychological, emotional, economic, social or legal. If a research problem involves a potentially harmful intervention, it may have to be abandoned, or at least restated to ensure it meets ethical requirements. For example, it would be unethical for a researcher to manipulate cigarette and alcohol consumption in a pregnant participant in order to observe the effects of substance abuse on the fetus and newborn. Before a study is conducted a review committee should decide whether data can be obtained from other sources, or by means of research methods other than one in which there is anticipated harm to the participant.

Although qualitative research is regarded as 'non-invasive' because it involves neither intervention nor treatment, qualitative researchers become involved in participants' lives for the duration of the study. A researcher should always use good judgement in the management of interviews. They should structure questions carefully and monitor participants for signs of distress. Should distress occur, the researcher must facilitate debriefing by giving participants the opportunity to ask questions or air complaints and, if necessary, refer them for counselling (Polit & Beck, 2021). Because participants enter into a special relationship with the researcher, additional care should be taken not to exploit this relationship. In qualitative research the development of a pseudo-therapeutic relationship may occur, causing additional risk to the participant. Care must be taken to always 'do good'. However, qualitative researchers may be in a good position to 'do good' by virtue of the specific participant–researcher relationship that they have with the participants.

Although research benefits society, institutions and individuals, it can also harm them. A neglected aspect of beneficence in research is that of reputational risk to the institution from which the study population is selected, as well as the institution undertaking the research. The researcher needs to be particularly careful not to identify the institution or community – in the report or any publication based on the report – to such an extent that its image or reputation could be damaged or brought into disrepute.

The participant is in a special relationship with the researcher and may not be exploited. The relationship is between the participant and a researcher and not the participant and a healthcare practitioner, manager or educator. Therefore, consent must result from an understanding of the researcher's role, not any other role. Participants may not be placed at a disadvantage. For example, in a study on drug abuse amongst students the participants must be assured that they will be protected should they divulge illegal practices such as drug trading.

Principle of justice

The principle of justice refers to a participant's right to fair selection and treatment and the right to privacy. Researchers must select a study's participants fairly for reasons directly related to the research problem. Researchers need to respect and honour any agreements they make with participants. If data needs to be collected through interviews, for example, the researcher should respect cultural values and terminate the process at the agreed time. Should a participant wish to withdraw from the study, no penalty may be imposed (directly or indirectly) nor may they be disadvantaged in any way.

Participants' privacy rights also need to be upheld. The participant has the right to determine the extent to and circumstances under which their private information is shared. Such information includes a participant's attitudes, beliefs, behaviour, opinions and medical records. A researcher who gathers data from participants without their knowledge – by recording conversations, observing activities through one-way mirrors and using hidden cameras and microphones, for example – invades participants' privacy. Participants' rights to privacy are also violated when a researcher shares information without their knowledge or against their will.

A research participant has the right to expect that information collected from or about them will remain anonymous and confidential. The researcher must therefore keep participants' identities secret. In fact, the researcher should not be able to link a participant with their data. For example, by distributing questionnaires and requesting that they be returned without any identifying details, the researcher ensures anonymity. If the results are to be published, the researcher must assure participants of the safeguards in place to protect their identities. This is particularly important when there is a small number of participants and the research setting is easily identifiable.

Research designed to collect data only once presents few problems in terms of anonymity. In this case, participant identification is unnecessary as there is only one set of responses. By contrast, research designed to compare individual performance over time presents a challenge to ensuring participant anonymity because the researcher may have to conduct follow-up interviews and will need a list of participants. The researcher should therefore be particularly careful about implementing and maintaining appropriate confidentiality procedures.

In situations such as focus-group interviews absolute anonymity is not possible. One rather aims at confidentiality binding agreements between and among the participants in the focus groups. When publishing case studies, for instance, the researcher may have to change some of the information so that participants are not easily identifiable.

The researcher can use any of the following mechanisms to ensure anonymity:
- provide participants with a number or code names or have them devise their own
- use code names when discussing data

- keep a list of participants' names and matching code names in a secure location
- destroy the list of participants' real names.

The process of ensuring confidentiality refers to a researcher's responsibility to prevent data from being linked to participants or being divulged for purposes other than research. If information is published, the researcher must inform participants and assure them that their anonymity will be maintained. All data, whether constituting responses to questionnaires or video- and audio-taped interviews (and transcriptions thereof), should be kept in a secure location.

Confidentiality breaches occur when researchers allow unauthorised persons access to data, or when they reveal participants' identities in reporting or publishing research findings. However, the researcher must plan for legitimate requests by institutions and other researchers in the field to use their research findings. They thus need to ensure that these scenarios are considered when they seek a participant's consent to partake in their study.

Procedures and mechanisms for protecting human rights

The researcher can use various procedures and mechanisms to ensure that participants' human rights are protected.

Informed consent

The ethical principles of voluntary participation and protecting the participants from harm are formalised in informed consent (Polit & Beck, 2022). This consent means that the participant has adequate information about the study, understands the information, and can consent to it or decline participation. The concept has three major elements:

1. the type of information needed from research participants
2. the degree of understanding participants must have to grant consent
3. the fact that participants choose whether or not to grant consent.

Information

In order to obtain participants' consent, the researcher must provide them with comprehensive information regarding their participation. Consent can be provided as follows:

- **written consent,** which is the preferred form of consent
- **implied consent,** where the submission of a completed self-administered questionnaire implies consent
- **process consent,** which takes place in qualitative research where repeated data collection takes place and it is difficult to obtain meaningful consent at the outset; this form of consent is negotiated continuously
- **verbal** consent
- **recorded** consent (audio or video recording).

The researcher selects an appropriate method after careful consideration of the participants' cognitive ability (to what extent are they literate?) and developmental level (what is the best way to present the information? Is the participant a child or an adult?) or based on the research approach.

Some research ethics committees (RECs) have strict formats with which the informed consent letter should comply. In many instances verbal, recorded or implied consent is not acceptable. The consent letter usually contains the following information:

- the research project's title
- an introduction to the research activities and an invitation to the participant to participate in the study
- the researcher's title and position (to enhance the credibility of the study)
- the project's purpose (including its long-term purpose)
- the selection criteria of the study population and sample (this indicates the population sample to be studied, as well as how and why they were selected)
- an explanation of data collection methods and procedures
- a description of risks and discomfort involved – be they physical, psychological, emotional, economic or social – as well as any benefits
- the benefits of participation to the participant
- suggestions of alternatives where a study involves an intervention or treatment
- a confirmation of anonymity and confidentiality (the term 'anonymous' should be used with caution, though, and never used if only confidentiality is possible)
- the voluntary nature of participation: participants must sign a non-coercive disclaimer, which states that participation is voluntary and that a refusal to participate will not involve any penalties; they must also be assured that they may withdraw at any time without any risks to their well-being
- the time that the research will require
- any costs involved for the participant
- consent to incomplete disclosure: where full disclosure could harm the study's validity, the participant should know that the researcher will deliberately withhold some information
- the researcher's offer to answer any questions
- a contact person's details
- clearly delineated spaces for the signatures of the researcher, the participant and a witness.

An example of an informed consent form appears in Figure 3.1. In many cases the signature of a witness is not required. The decision lies with the particular REC.

EATING PATTERNS SUCCESSFUL DIETERS USE
TO MAINTAIN WEIGHT LOSS

INVESTIGATOR: PATRICIA MBOMBO
RN.MN

Dear _____

Thank you for responding to the advertisement in the Morning Star requesting information from successful dieters. I hereby invite you to participate in my study. The purpose of the research is to determine whether there are common features in the personal histories of successful dieters that can be shared with those who have been unsuccessful in their weight loss goals. Although the study will not benefit you directly, the information obtained may help those who have trouble losing weight and maintaining weight loss to hear how you (and other successful dieters) were able to lose weight. | Purpose / Potential benefit

There are no risks involved in sharing your story. You will be required to meet with me once for a voice-recorded interview lasting approximately an hour. A photograph of yourself when overweight, or in an item of clothing you may have saved, will also be required. Furthermore, I will need to weigh you on my calibrated scale and measure your height. | Risks / Time commitment

I shall keep a record of the study's participants, as well as recordings of our interviews (together with a transcription of those recordings). Your name will not appear on the recording or transcriptions, and that information will not be linked to you. All data will be stored in a secure place and no one, except the research team, will have access to it. In addition, your identity will not be revealed when the study is reported or published. | Explanation of procedures / Anonymity / Confidentiality

Your participation in this study is totally voluntary and you are under no obligation to participate. You can withdraw at any time without repercussion or penalty, even in the middle of an interview. | Voluntary consent and option to withdraw

This study and its procedures have been approved by the appropriate individuals and research committees of the university. | Board or committee approval

I have discussed the points above with the participant, and it is my opinion that they understand the risks, benefits and obligations involved in participating in this project.

_____   _____
Investigator   Date

I understand that my participation in this study is voluntary. I know that I can refuse to participate and/or withdraw my consent at any time without penalty.

If you have any questions about the study or about participating in the study, please feel free to contact me (Patricia Mbombo). You can call me at 011 111 2222 (work) or 012 222 3333 (home). | Offer to answer questions

_____   _____   _____
Signature of witness   Signature of participant   Date

Figure 3.1 An informed consent form template

Understanding

The information contained in the informed consent communication needs to be understood by the participant. It should therefore be in the participant's own language, pitched at the correct level and not contain technical language or jargon.

The researcher can determine whether the participant understands the requirements of the study by asking them questions. Participants sometimes need to think about their participation and return with questions. Confirmation of consent can take place when both parties agree that each understands their requirements.

Choice

The researcher is responsible for ensuring that the participant is not unduly influenced or coerced into participation. A prospective participant has to decide whether or not to participate and must be given time to consider their decision. They must feel confident that their refusal will not prejudice them in any way.

Voluntary consent is obtained only once the participant demonstrates a clear understanding of the informed consent form. Most procedures which need informed consent are based on experimental studies. In longitudinal studies and qualitative research, informed consent is an ongoing process. The researcher should re-obtain the participant's informed consent (a process known as 'process consent') as the study develops because unexpected events could occur and new research questions may emerge.

Issues relating to informed consent

Although researchers endorse the participants' rights to self-determination and informed consent, certain issues and circumstances make these standards difficult to uphold. One of the main issues is the inability to make informed decisions. Vulnerable groups (like children, or those who are mentally or intellectually challenged) may be incapable of providing informed consent. In these cases the researcher must obtain proxy consent. In all cases the researcher should make absolutely sure that the risks are as low as possible in comparison to the possible benefit.

In the case of children, parents or legal guardians should grant permission. This process is based on each country's legislation related to children participating in research. However, if the child is able to comprehend what the research entails, they must also provide assent. Assent refers to the affirmative agreement of a vulnerable individual, such as a child, to participate in a study to supplement the formal consent by a parent or legal guardian (Polit & Beck, 2022).

In certain situations, the researcher cannot inform participants about every aspect of a procedure as this could negate the treatment effects. For example, the reaction of a group of students to a crisis may be artificial if they know that the crisis is being staged in order to gauge their reactions. In a case like this the researcher may withhold information or provide them with false information.

Burns and Grove (2020) argue that the use of deception must be dealt with carefully. If deception is used in a study, it is important to explain in the report how the participants were deceived and how they were informed of the deception and the actual research activities (thus providing full information) after the study was completed. While some researchers argue that the use of deception is never justified, others believe that if the study exposes participants to minimal risk, if there are anticipated benefits to science and society, and if there are no other research alternatives, then the method may be justified. Babbie and Mouton (2021), for instance, argue that there is no reason why participants cannot be informed afterwards and recommend that they should be informed. When deception is deemed necessary for the purposes of research, participants need to be debriefed. That is, the researcher must inform the participants of the reasons, discuss with them any misconceptions, and attempt to remove any harmful effects of the process.

Researchers must train fieldworkers to obtain voluntary informed consent to ensure understanding and to respect the dignity and individuality of all participants. Fieldworkers and co-investigators must also sign a confidentiality agreement (also referred to as confidentiality binding form) before they can join the research team. In lengthy or international multi-site studies, attention must be given to the informed consent process and to understanding cultural and religious values as well as country-specific requirements related to research ethics. Depending on the risk level, renewal of consent after a specific period may be required by the research ethics boards.

It is recommended that researchers study the guidelines laid out in the South African Department of Health's 2015 edition of *Ethics in Health Research: Principles, Processes and Structures*. The guidelines are intended for use by researchers who involve human participants in their research. The guidelines cover the following:
- the minimum national benchmark of norms and standards
- a detailed explication of the process of ethics review and focused guidance about specific topics and research methodologies
- the expectations and standards for Research Ethics Committees (RECs) and Animal Research Ethics Committees and guidance about standard operating procedures
- the research ethics infrastructure and regulatory framework in South Africa.

The risk–benefit ratio

Before a study commences, researchers and reviewers of research must examine the ratio of benefit to risk involved. The benefits are the positive values that the research provides, and include a study's potential contribution to knowledge, its practical value to society and its use to participants. Risks refer to the possibility that participants may be harmed during the research process. While all research involves a certain amount of risk, the general guideline is that risk should not exceed potential benefits. When risk is high the researcher must make every effort to reduce it and to maximise benefits instead. Should the risks outweigh the benefits, the study should not be undertaken.

Potential **benefits** include:

- increased knowledge about healthcare practices or a participant's condition
- improvement in the participant's understanding of healthcare delivery
- enhanced self-esteem in the participant because of the special attention they have been given
- participants' rapid recovery from illness
- improvement in healthcare delivery to the public
- improved health needs assessments
- increased understanding of preventive health measures.

Potential **risks** include:

- physical harm to the participant in the form of unanticipated side-effects (in the case of serious unanticipated side-effects, the study should be stopped immediately and reported to the relevant ethics committee)
- physical discomfort, fatigue or boredom on the part of the participant
- psychological or emotional distress in the participant, resulting from self-disclosure, introspection, fear of the unknown and/or fear of repercussions
- privacy loss or violation on the part of the participant
- financial costs.

The obligation to ensure benefits outweigh risks is not only the responsibility of the researcher, though – other professionals and society are also accountable. Professionals must be members of research boards and committees in order to ensure ethical research is conducted, and society needs to be involved in research enterprises and must concern itself with the protection of participants (Gray, Grove & Sutherland, 2017; Moodley, 2017).

Risks are categorised as follows:

- Category 1: Negligible risk – No or indirect human participant involvement.
- Category 2: Low risk – Direct human participant involvement. The only foreseeable risk of harm is the potential for minor discomfort or inconvenience, thus research would not pose a risk above the everyday norm.
- Category 3: Medium risk – Direct human participant involvement. Research poses a risk above the everyday norm, including physical, psychological and social risks. Steps can be taken to minimise the likelihood of the event occurring.
- Category 4: High risk – Direct human participant involvement. There is a real or foreseeable risk of harm including physical, psychological and social risk that may lead to a serious adverse event if not managed responsibly.

Scientific honesty and other responsibilities

In addition to honouring the rights of participants, researchers must demonstrate respect for the scientific community by protecting the integrity of scientific knowledge. Researchers have ethical responsibilities associated with the conduct and reporting of research. They must be competent, ensure accuracy and, above all, be honest in everything they do.

It is also essential for researchers to manage resources – whether financial, human or material – in an effective, efficient and economical manner. Poorly planned and conducted research is likely to be ineffective and inefficient and is unethical. Researchers also need to obtain permission to conduct their studies from the relevant authorities, employers and/or owners of the institutions, premises or materials they intend to use.

To maintain research integrity, the researcher must avoid the following activities:

- **Fabrication, falsification or forgery.** The researcher cannot invent information, nor compile a report that does not reflect what they actually did.
- **Manipulation of design and methods.** The researcher cannot plan the design and data-collection methods of the study to ensure results will support their viewpoints.
- **Selective retention and/or manipulation of data.** The researcher cannot choose to use only the data which supports their viewpoints and discard the rest, nor manipulate data to reflect their perspective.
- **Plagiarism.** The researcher cannot present the work or ideas of someone else as their own.
- **Irresponsible collaboration.** When appointed a member of a research team, the researcher cannot participate inappropriately or not fulfil their responsibilities.

The ever-changing nature of technology has also affected research and research practices. In addition, global health patterns such as the Covid-19 pandemic brought about evolving changes in research. Online research is becoming inseparable from our lives as researchers and practitioners. We are redefining ways that ethical research practices apply when we use information-communication technologies to collect and analyse data and disseminate findings. Therefore, ethical principles and concepts are also reconsidered and redefined to suit the current trends. It should also be noted that while the internet can be used to conduct research using tools like SurveyMonkey and social media polls, issues such as privacy, confidentiality and whether parental assent is required still need consideration. The ethical issues involved in these forms of research are complicated and differ according to international legislation about participants' rights to privacy. Many of these issues are currently under investigation and researchers need to bear them in mind when developing strategies to protect participants from privacy violations (Gray et al, 2017; Salmons, 2016).

Ethics review boards and committees

In addition to codes of research and ethical guidelines, most institutions have established independent committees to review research proposals and to examine and monitor ethical standards of ongoing research. These committees are referred to as 'institutional review boards' (IRBs), research ethics committees (RECs), 'ethics committees' or 'research committees'. Researchers must submit their research proposals along with the necessary consent forms to the appropriate committee(s) for review before the commencement of a project. Authors of scientific articles will be required to provide ethics certificates or project numbers before their research can be published in scientific journals.

Every researcher – from undergraduate student to seasoned professional – must be aware of the ethical rules and regulations governing research at their institution and must obtain clearance before embarking on data collection. Ethical clearance may also be required from the research setting's ethical review board. This is of particular importance if a study is registered in one country and data collection is conducted in another country because of the research setting. This is often the case where international students who study in South Africa conduct the research in their home country.

The role of ethics review boards and committees

The submission of research proposals for review by a committee is a procedure which protects the researcher and the research participants. The committee members consider every aspect of the proposal, including its ethical aspects. They may reject it outright or recommend changes if they are not satisfied that it adheres to established scientific and ethical guidelines. The ethics review boards also carefully consider the risk level categories to ensure that participants are always protected.

Research studies may be exempted from review, which means that they are not subjected to a full review by an ethics review board. This category is referred to as negligible risk studies and includes various types of reviews (e g systematic, integrative, scoping reviews). In studies where there are no apparent risks for the research participant, like those dealing with observations of public behaviour that do not identify participants or place them at risk, and studies which make use of publicly available data, such as artefacts, photographs and historical documents, a full ethics review may also not be required. However, the responsibility of the researcher to protect the participants does not change.

Evaluation of the ethical elements of a research proposal or report

You may be called upon to serve on a research committee or review board, or to assess the research proposals or reports of peers. In the same way that a research proposal must be ethically acceptable to be approved, ethical implications are also important if you are adopting research findings in practice. An ethical committee's checklist is one guide you can use to review a report.

However, reports do not always provide detailed information regarding the degree to which the researcher adhered to ethical principles because of space limitations in professional journals. But even without detailed descriptions you can evaluate various facets of the report from an ethical perspective. You can ask the following questions:

- Is the research problem significant?
- Is the design scientifically sound?
- Is the research designed to maximise benefits and minimise risks?
- Are appropriate steps in place to prevent physical harm or psychological distress?
- Is participant selection ethical?

- Is there evidence of voluntary informed consent? If not, is there a valid and justifiable reason why this aspect has not been included?
- Has informed consent been given by the legal guardian or representative of a participant incapable of providing their own consent? Is there evidence of assent in cases of vulnerable groups such as minor children?
- Is there evidence of deception?
- Have appropriate steps been taken to safeguard the participant's privacy?

Summary

In this chapter we presented in detail the need for professional ethical guidelines in conducting health sciences research. We explored the rights of the participants as well as the ways in which researchers can protect those rights, how participants are selected and invited to participate in the study, what information they must be given, what choice they have, how confidentiality and anonymity will be maintained, what risks have been identified and how to minimise them while maximising the benefits. We considered scientific honesty. The chapter closed with a discussion of the role of ethics review boards and committees and provided a set of guidelines that a member of such a board or committee can use to evaluate the ethical implications of a research report.

Exercises

1. Read the National Health Act 61 of 2003 in relation to research ethics. Summarise the important research-related guidelines provided by the Act.

2. Identify three examples where research would be unethical based on the stipulations of the Act.

3. Search for two recent and relevant articles online using the search terms 'decolonisation and research ethics' and 'research and indigenous communities'. Read the articles and highlight the specific ethical principles related to research with indigenous communities.

4. A researcher plans to investigate second-year students' knowledge and skills in a crisis that arose after a flood disaster. She wants to observe reactions to the crisis as they occur. She thus does not reveal the exact nature of the study to the participants. Each student is instructed to measure the anxiety levels of a patient as part of the patient's continuous assessment. The patient – a volunteer who has been briefed by the researcher – simulates a panic attack while the student is doing the assessment. A research assistant observes the timeliness and

⮕

appropriateness of the students' responses through a one-way mirror. Immediately afterwards, the students are debriefed and paid R100 for their participation.

(a) Discuss the ethical implications of conducting this study with an emphasis on vulnerability, risk–benefit ratio, and the participants' rights to self-determination and privacy. Was there a justifiable reason for the researcher not having obtained informed consent before conducting the study?

(b) What type of participants' review would be appropriate for this study?

(c) Describe any debriefing information the study should include.

Here are some websites you may find useful:

- National Research Foundation: http://www.nrf.ac.za
- Oxford Handbooks Online DOI: 10.1093/oxfordhb/9780190947750.013.47
- American Nurses Association Code of Ethics for Nurses – http://www.ana. org/ – you can follow the links from 'Nursing Ethics' to the 'Code of Ethics for Nurses'
- Human Sciences Research Council (South Africa): http://www.hsrc.ac.za/ en/about/research-ethics/code-of-research-ethics
- Council for International Organizations of Medical Sciences (CIOMS) in collaboration with the World Health Organization (WHO). 2016. http:// www.cioms.ch/index.php/12-newsflash/403-new-cioms-international-ethical-guidelines-now-available

An overview of the research process

Chapter 4

> **LEARNING OUTCOMES**
>
> On completion of this chapter, you should be able to demonstrate your understanding of:
> - the major phases of the research process
> - the steps of the research process that are likely to occur in each phase
> - a practical model of the research process in health sciences
> - a variety of models of the research process in health sciences
> - a research setting

This chapter presents a general overview of the research process. Later chapters discuss each phase and step in greater detail. The research process presented here is a model: it provides a representation of reality. Therefore, the phases presented in an orderly fashion here do not necessarily reflect the way they play out in real-life scenarios. While some phases may occur concurrently, the researcher can work on more than one step at a time or may omit one and return to it later. Whatever the order selected, the researcher should address the phases in a systematic manner. Research sources differ regarding the number of phases, which can be anything from four to eight. For the purpose of this book we describe the research process as a four-phased process. We do, however, also show examples where the process is described as having more phases.

The research process

Research is a dynamic process that can be organised into four stages: *Exploring, Investigating, Processing,* and *Creating*. As you work through a research project, you may move back and forth between these stages as your understanding evolves. Research is a process which begins with a problem and ends with that problem being resolved or addressed. Research stimulates further research and cannot be seen as a once-off, linear or static act.

The research process consists of four interactive, but broad, phases:
1. The **conceptual phase**, which is also known as the 'thinking' or 'planning phase'. The standard elements of this phase are the research problem and the research question, which are always preceded by a literature review to determine what is already known.
2. The **empirical phase**, also called the 'doing phase'. The standard element is research design.

3. The **interpretive phase** (where the researcher engages with the meaning of the study). The standard element is empirical evidence.
4. The **communication phase**. This is writing up the research report and disseminating findings for both publication and knowledge translation. The standard element is the set of conclusions.

Each phase can be divided into steps which hinge on a study's purpose as well as its research approach and design. While the number of steps remains a contentious issue (and varies from 8 to 17), it is essential that the research process follows logical and scientific conventions to address the problem identified.

Although Table 4.1 lists 11 steps, you may have to adapt this model to the specific needs of your research. If adaptations are made, you must clearly motivate your change(s), and demonstrate that you have considered and recorded the implications for the research process as a whole and the participants in particular.

Table 4.1 Steps in the research process

1. Identify the problem and the research question. 2. Determine the purpose of the study. 3. Review related literature and develop a theoretical or conceptual framework. 4. Define and refine the research question and formulate a research hypothesis. 5. Select the research method and determine the design of the study. 6. Specify the group of elements to be studied.	Phase 1 – Conceptual
7. Conduct a pilot study. 8. Collect the data.	Phase 2 – Empirical
9. Analyse the data. 10. Interpret the results.	Phase 3 – Interpretive
11. Communicate the research findings.	Phase 4 – Communication

The steps outlined above are interdependent and interrelated – reflecting both the varying amounts of detail included and the different ways of categorising specific research activities. They are most suited to a quantitative approach. Should a qualitative approach be used, the researcher will follow step 3 later in the research process as part of the literature control and integration. However, some qualitative researchers follow step 3 in the form of a scoping narrative or integrative review. The researcher would also not follow step 4 exactly as is because one is not concerned with testing a hypothesis in qualitative research.

Major phases and steps in the research process

We provide an outline of the major phases and steps in this section. In following chapters more detail is provided on the specific steps that are to be followed.

Phase 1: The conceptual phase

Research normally begins with phase one, which typically involves the process of 'conceptualisation' – that is, the development and refinement of abstract ideas. During this phase, the researcher categorises and labels their impressions while involved in activities which include thinking, reading, rethinking, theorising, making decisions about ideas, and reviewing ideas which draw on creativity, analysis and insight, as well as on the firm grounding of existing research on the topic of interest.

Step 1: Identify the problem and the research question

A research project begins with a problem and a good research question and is key to the researcher's decisions about design, data collection and analysis. The research problem is a statement about an area of concern, a condition or a situation that needs change, a difficulty to be addressed, or a troubling question identified from scientific and scholarly theory, literature or practice. A research problem thus relates to the gap found in the knowledge which needs to be addressed. Without a sound and viable research problem and research question, even the most carefully and skilfully designed project is of little value. Problems and research questions originate from a variety of sources such as personal experience, issues in communities or organisations, clinical settings in healthcare, and problems presented in literature or theories. Researchers generally proceed from a broad topic area to a specific set of questions or objectives that will address the identified problem.

The research problem:
- indicates the significance of the problem
- provides a background for the problem
- includes a problem statement, which could be formulated in either a declarative statement or an interrogative form (question form).

Step 2: Determine the purpose of the study

The research purpose is derived from the problem and aims to answer the research question. It identifies the study's specific goal and describes the scope of the research. It is a clear and concise statement of the specific goal or focus of the study. The researcher may identify, describe, investigate, explain or predict a solution to the problem, evaluate a practice or programme, or develop an instrument. In a qualitative study the purpose might be to explore and describe a phenomenon, develop strategies, guidelines, a theory or model, or describe historical events or patterns.

Step 3: Review related literature and develop a theoretical or conceptual framework

The literature review identifies what is known and not known about the research problem. The researcher must conduct a literature review to locate existing studies which may serve as a basis for theirs. The literature review assists the researcher in developing a theoretical or conceptual framework, and allows them to select appropriate methods, instruments and tools with which to measure the study's variables.

The review should be comprehensive and must cover all relevant research and supporting documents in print (ie textbooks, reports, journal articles, theses, dissertations, periodical and citation indexes) and online resources. A thorough review of related literature requires time and effort, and computer-generated searches can assist tremendously with this process. Although seldom done since the development of electronic databases, hardcopy textual investigations should not be dismissed, as libraries have access to sources which may not be indexed or available in electronic databases. The assistance of a librarian can also be a valuable resource.

Occasionally the initial review of the literature (sometimes called a rapid review) may precede the identification of the problem as the researcher's conceptual insights and ideas regarding topics, approaches or techniques are stimulated. The review is guided by a search strategy, which includes a question, search terms, publication type, period published, language preference and exclusionary criteria. A review with a well-planned search strategy renders more relevant and appropriate references.

Step 4: Define and refine the research question and formulate a research hypothesis

A research problem is identified through the researcher's observation, knowledge, wisdom and skills. In this step the researcher must construct the research problem in a manner which facilitates further research. The problem should be measurable and generate or refine essential knowledge. The researcher thus moves from a broad, abstractly stated problem and purpose to specific objectives, questions or hypotheses. These should provide a specific focus which must be clearly stated. For example: 'The purpose is to explore the experiences regarding visiting rights of family members of a Covid-19 patient in a critical care unit', or 'What are the multiple HIV risk factors associated with female sex workers?' In the latter case the researcher may have found information suggesting that associated factors such as gender-based violence affect the exposure to risk factors. The hypothesis could be: 'Sex workers experiencing gender-based violence from multiple perpetrators are more exposed to HIV risk factors than those who do not experience gender-based violence.'

Step 5: Select the research method and determine the design of the study

The research design ensures that the research problem is addressed effectively and constitutes the blueprint for the methods that will be used. This step entails the researcher designing the study. The choice of design depends on the researcher's expertise, the problem, and the purpose of the study. It must also take into account previous well-designed studies and the researcher's desire to generalise the findings. The researcher needs to decide on the following:

- **Approach** – which research approach (quantitative, qualitative) will best answer the research question and meet the objectives? Which design (eg a descriptive design, case study, experiment, ethnographic study, phenomenological study or historical study) is best? In a mixed methods design both approaches will be used in different order and varying levels of dominance and order. Considerations must include permissions which may be required, ethical dilemmas, the timing of each step and how terminology is defined. Research sources differ in the use of terms describing the research approach. Some sources refer to 'research paradigms', 'strategies' or 'research design'. For the purposes of this book, we refer to 'research approaches' when describing the qualitative and quantitative approaches to a study.
- **Population and sample** – who will constitute the study population? Which population is accessible and can be represented best? Which criteria are to be used in sample selection, and in decisions concerning sample size and method of contact?
- **Instrument** – that is, which procedure should be used to gather data? Should one or more instruments be used in data collection? Should an existing instrument be used? Which instrument will yield the most significant information? Will the instrument yield reliable and valid information? Will one need to develop a new questionnaire? What type of data should the instrument generate – for example, numerical or non-numerical?
- **Data-collection procedure (protocol)** – which consists of the various procedures for collecting information. The researcher must consider the advantages and disadvantages of each, as well as what the time and financial constraints about, for example, travel and actual collection of data will be. How will data collection commence?
- **Data-analysis plan** – what is to be done with the data once they have been gathered?

Step 6: Specify the group of elements to be studied

The researcher must decide who or what can render the data needed to answer the research question. Individuals are known as 'research participants', while the 'population' refers to all the elements – that is, individuals, objects, events or substances – which meet the criteria for inclusion in an identified universe. The definition of 'population' depends on the sample criteria and the similarity of elements in these settings. The researcher must determine which population is accessible and can be best represented by the study sample. It is not always possible for the researcher to study all elements: instead, they must use a sample. The researcher will have to finalise the criteria to be used in the selection of the sample, decide how to ensure its representativeness, and select the sampling method as well as the sample size.

Phase 2: The empirical phase

The empirical phase enables the researcher to observe or measure phenomena, as directly experienced by the researcher. In this phase the researcher implements the data collection plans made in phase 1. A well-planned phase 1 is thus critical because any shortcomings could affect scientific rigour in all the other phases. The empirical phase is often the most time-consuming.

Step 7: Conduct a pilot study

Until this point only conceptual decision-making and planning has taken place, but the researcher is now ready to implement the plan. Where possible, though, they should first conduct a pilot study – a small-scale version, or 'dummy run', of the main study. Since unforeseen problems can arise during the course of a project, a pilot study allows the researcher to recognise and address some of them and means that they can make adjustments to the main study.

The pilot study is sometimes viewed as part of the planning phase, as it may bring about changes before data collection commences. In some studies the pilot study is omitted in favour of a data-collection instrument pre-test. Pre-testing the instrument allows for its refinement and is done where a complete pilot study is not conducted. It is good practice for qualitative researchers to do a pre-test of the interview process where the researcher's interviewing skills, the location where the interview will be conducted and the functioning of the audio-recorder are tested to ensure the flow and conduct of the interviews will be in order. Should data be collected using online methods, such as through Teams or Skype, the connectivity, software program and its functionality are tested.

Step 8: Collect the data

The researcher usually collects data in accordance with the pre-established plan using the instrument developed and tested in the pilot study or pre-test. If the study participants have not yet been selected, this aspect needs to be addressed at this point. The researcher contacts the participants to explain the study to them and to obtain their consent. Once the research proposal has been finalised, institutions, authorities or agencies where the study is conducted usually grant permission for the study to be conducted. In some instances, especially in cross-country studies, ethical clearance must be sought from the relevant ethical clearance committees. An example would be where a study is approved in South Africa, but conducted in hospitals in Ethiopia. Ethical clearance must then also be sought from the Ethiopian Ministry of Health before the study can commence. In cases of multiple country studies, ethical clearance will be required from all participating countries or institutions (depending on the requirements and proposal format of each country).

The data collection methods vary according to the research design. The researcher may observe, question or measure the most frequently used methods, and use instruments such as observations, interviews, questionnaires or scales. Meaningful research demands that each piece of data has a purpose related to the study's goal.

Phase 3: The interpretive phase

The data collected in the empirical phase are not reported in 'raw' form: the researcher must summarise the information or enter the data in a database and subject it to various types of analysis and interpretation.

Step 9: Analyse the data

Before analysing or processing the data the researcher must examine them for completeness and accuracy. Incomplete and inaccurately completed questionnaires are usually discarded. However, in some instances the data is used with specific reference to missing values. The researcher must then organise the data in an orderly, coherent fashion in order to discern patterns and relationships. Narrative data is transcribed word for word to enable the researcher to commence with the coding of the data.

The process of data analysis is determined by the research approach because researchers analyse quantitative and qualitative data differently. Analysis techniques used in quantitative research include descriptive and inferential statistics and advanced analysis (processes which are usually automated). Qualitative analysis involves the integration and synthesis of narrative non-numeric data which are reduced to themes and categories with the aid of a coding procedure. Thus, a descriptive design, an experiment and a grounded theory study will all produce different types and amounts of data. In mixed methods research the data sets are analysed based on the specific procedures and processes, after which all data sets are integrated.

Step 10: Interpret the results

The results obtained from data analysis require interpretation (the researcher's act of drawing conclusions and making sense of the results) for them to be meaningful.

As part of the process, the researcher asks the following questions:

- What do the results imply?
- Were the objectives or research questions addressed?
- What can be learned from the data?
- What do the findings mean for others in similar contexts?
  - What is the value of the study for them?
  - How do the findings compare to the findings of other studies?
  - Should the study encourage changes to their policies?
  - Should the study encourage change in their assumptions about issues like curricula or practice?
- What recommendations can be made for further research?
- What limitation did the findings yield?

Phase 4: The communication phase

In phase 3 the researcher answers the questions posed in phase 1. However, the job is not complete until the researcher communicates the study's results to others. During this phase the research results become public knowledge.

Step 11: Communicate the research findings

The research process is incomplete without a scientific research report. Communicating findings involves the development and dissemination of a research report to appropriate audiences in a suitable language and format. The key is to *effectively* communicate the findings. The report must reflect each step of the process and indicate the final product. It should be well organised, informative and succinct. For an executive summary or a broad overview to management, a 'one-pager' is often all that is required. Management does not always require a full report. Sometimes the executive summary provides the focused overview required during decision-making. In such cases we talk about knowledge translation, the activities involved in translating or moving research from the research setting to the institutions and individuals who will put the recommendations into practice. It is a dynamic and an iterative process that assists in the understanding of how to implement research to improve practice and policy and address risks and benefits to make informed decisions. One example of a model for knowledge translation is 'The knowledge-to-action framework', which provides a model for the promotion of the application of research and the process of knowledge translation. You can research 'knowledge translation' to learn more about this.

Researchers should familiarise themselves with the publication policies of journals. In their report researchers must convey the study's findings in an intelligible manner and their writing style should be appropriate for the publication's readers. The correct technical presentation of the research report contributes to the scientific value of the study and must be adhered to. Here the scientific integrity of the researcher is of utmost importance – results and findings must not be falsified or fabricated, but should be a true reflection of what was discovered in the study. Plagiarism must be prevented and correct and sufficient referencing of sources must be maintained.

Other additional ways of communicating research findings are oral or poster presentations at conferences, presenting a webinar or workshop, or publishing abstracts, short research reports or briefs and journal articles.

Other models of the research process

Researchers and studies differ in terms of process and procedures. As a researcher one must make a decision on how to best follow a scientific process in completing a study. The following models are similar to the model presented above, although they differ in the number of phases and/or steps. Should you be interested in using one of the models below, use the relevant and corresponding information on each step as discussed earlier in this chapter.

Polit and Beck (2004; 2021) describe five phases to the research process: the *conceptual phase*, the *design and planning phase*, the *empirical phase*, the *analytic phase*, and the *dissemination phase*.

Model using five steps

- Step 1 – Locating and defining issues or problems. This step focuses on uncovering the nature and boundaries of a situation or question that needs to be answered or studied.
- Step 2 – Designing the research project
- Step 3 – Collecting data
- Step 4 – Interpreting research data
- Step 5 – Report research findings.

Model using eight steps

- Step 1 – Identify the problem
- Step 2 – Review literature
- Step 3 – Set research questions, objectives and hypotheses
- Step 4 – Choose the study design
- Step 5 – Decide on the sample design
- Step 6 – Collect data
- Step 7 – Process and analyse data
- Step 8 – Write the report.

Research setting

A 'research setting' refers to the specific place or places (site or location) where the data are collected. The decision about where a study is to be conducted is based on the research question and the type of data needed to address it. The setting needs to be clearly described and the selection justified. A naturalistic setting is an uncontrolled, real-life situation or environment. These settings may be participants' homes, clinical settings or educational settings. The researcher does not manipulate or change the environment. Qualitative researchers are especially likely to conduct research in such settings.

Research can also take place in a partially controlled or highly controlled setting, such as a laboratory. A partially controlled setting is an environment which has been partially manipulated or modified by the researcher. This type of setting tends to be used more frequently because the researcher can limit the effects of extraneous variables on the study's outcome. For example, where two groups of students are part of a study on academic performance, the researcher would keep the groups in different rooms in order to limit the impact the environment has on the responses of the students. A highly controlled setting is developed specifically for research or testing and can include a laboratory, or a test centre or unit. Because the influence of extraneous variables is reduced, the effect of one variable on another can be accurately measured.

A 'research site' refers to the overall location for the research. A site could therefore refer to an entire university (such as a university in Cape Town), institution (such as a hospital in Johannesburg) or community (such as Bushbuck Ridge or Durban). Multisite studies could be undertaken using multiple sites as mentioned above.

Summary

In this chapter we provided an overview of the major phases and steps of the research process. The process was depicted as a model which, while giving an idealised view of reality, is nevertheless useful as a guide for the planning, implementation and monitoring of the research. The model divides the process into phases and steps, which assists the researcher in preparing a flexible schedule for the time to be spent on each phase. We presented the phases and steps sequentially, while pointing out and emphasising their interdependent and interrelated nature. The model presented in this chapter was particularly applicable to quantitative research and can be adjusted for qualitative studies. We also provided other models that have different phases and steps and could be used with the guidance of the information provided in this chapter.

Exercises

1. Read a research article that interests you. Can you identify the steps of the research process? If not, which are missing? Discuss the significance of the missing step or steps with your colleagues.

2. Compare a research article and an information article. Are you able to identify the differences? Describe the scientific value of both articles.

3. Select and describe a current public health problem in your country, and then outline the steps a researcher should take to study it.

4. Using a different example than in question 3, outline the steps a researcher could use to complete the study, selecting a different model with different steps.

5. If you were conducting research about the effect of online learning on academic performance, what would the various steps entail?

6. Using the example in question 5, outline the research setting and site, and justify your choice.

Selecting or identifying research problems

Chapter 4 explained that the first step in the first phase of the research process is the identification of a problem area or topic of interest. The research problem provides guidance for developing the research question(s), aims and objectives of the study. It is also the primary focus in a research report. Indeed, the researcher cannot conceptualise and implement a study without a clear, researchable problem.

What is a research topic?

A research topic – also referred to as a 'concept', the 'phenomenon of interest to the researcher' or the 'domain of inquiry' – acts as the basis for question generation or research purpose generation. In the health sciences the topic can be categorised according to several major areas:

- practice
- education
- policy
- health services management
- history
- ethics
- person- or situation-based variables.

A research topic is the research question one is going to answer. Funders and research institutions are structured to support the best resources, facilities and expertise to conduct research. Thus, a sound and viable research question improves the quality of healthcare for patients and healthcare professionals alike.

Before the researcher can identify the research problem, they need to answer the following questions:

- Am I interested enough in the topic to maintain my attentiveness for the duration of the study?
- Although a broad outline of the phenomenon, is the topic specific enough to be researched?
- Will the topic elicit a single interpretation so that others do not get distracted?
- Is the topic researchable in terms of time, resources and availability of data?
- Could the results of the study contribute to the health sciences' body of knowledge?
- Should I present the topic in the form of a dissertation, a research report or an article?
- Does the topic fall under an institution's or funder's focus?

Research problem and purpose

The research problem is an area of concern in which there is a gap or a situation in need of solution, improvement or alteration, or in which there is a discrepancy between the way things are and the way they ought to be. It therefore refers to a troubling situation. A researcher can identify a problem by asking the following questions:

- What is the cause for concern?
- How and why is this problem significant?
- Where is the knowledge gap situated?
- What interventions could work in a clinical situation?
- What changes could improve the situation?

A **research problem** can also originate from the researcher's interest in a topic: for example, a critical analysis of music therapy on patients in a coma, or an investigation into the use of storytelling as a teaching strategy for health sciences students. Some problems are more relevant to qualitative research and others may suit quantitative designs better. It is important that the research problem can be addressed by the research question(s) asked.

To clarify a research problem the researcher must perform a preliminary literature review and gain an understanding of the scope and impact of the problem. This process culminates in a **problem statement** that clearly states the gap or discrepancy on which the proposed study will focus (Grove, Gray & Burns, 2018).

The research purpose is generated from the problem and the research question. It clearly and concisely states the aim(s) of the study by way of 'exploring', 'describing', 'identifying' or 'predicting' a solution to the problem. The research purpose therefore captures the essence of the study in a single sentence, which also outlines the study's variables, population and research setting.

Origins of research problems

Research problems derive from sources such as clinical practice, literature, theory, ethical dilemmas, observed health and illness patterns, established research priorities, and interactions with colleagues, students, individuals and communities. Researchers often use more than one source.

Table 5.1 illustrates how each of these areas can influence idea generation for a research problem and lists their most common sources.

Table 5.1 The influence of selected sources on research idea development

Source	Influence	Example
Clinical practice	The healthcare professional may identify problem areas: • through observations • in patient assessment interactions • in interaction with others • in the application or implementation of treatment.	• A healthcare professional working in a surgical ward may observe that patients do not comply with wound care programmes once they are discharged, despite patient education programmes. They therefore recognise that patient compliance requires more attention. • A healthcare professional working in a clinic may observe a higher proportion of drug abuse among adolescents than they have noted in other communities. They may then identify drug abuse as a possible contextual problem area. • A healthcare professional working in a surgical ward may observe differences in the length of time needed for wounds to heal on patients with similar wounds (but who receive different dressings). They therefore recognise wound dressings as a problem area. • A healthcare professional working in a primary healthcare clinic observes that some of the patients (who all attended the same funeral) complain of similar symptoms shortly after the funeral. They want to investigate this observation.
Health sciences literature	The healthcare professional may find contradictory information or gaps in literature. The healthcare professional may also identify studies to replicate.	A healthcare professional in charge of an orthopaedic ward reads two articles on post-operative pain management using intravenous infiltration. One author recommends that the infiltration should be altered with oral pain medication, while the other recommends intravenous infiltration only. The question (problem area) is: which of the two methods is most effective for pain relief?

Source	Influence	Example
Theory	Theories such as Orem's self-care theory, people's interaction theory, stress theory, motivation theory etc, may form the basis for research. The health sciences researcher could ask: if theory x is correct, what are the implications for people's behaviours, or emotional states in certain situations?	A healthcare professional could explore a concept such as self-care in Orem's theory or investigate the success of motivation strategies.
Patient and key stakeholder involvement	Inputs from patients and key stakeholders such as allied health professionals or leaders in health-related fields assist in identifying important issues for research. Patient-centred outcomes research has become prominent.	A healthcare professional could explore the needs of older persons to make an informed choice about the visiting times of family members in a sub-acute unit at a care institution for older persons.
Quality improvement initiatives	Involvement in quality improvement committees can sometimes lead to ideas for further studies. Root cause analysis can lead to and suggest a research focus.	A study could be conducted that investigates the best practices to improve student support at a distance education institution.
Social issues	Social and political issues may influence healthcare. Public awareness about healthcare disparities has often led to researchable questions. Cultural sensitivity in terms of healthcare provision may require new interventions.	A researcher could investigate cultural-sensitive care in terms of personal female care.

Source	Influence	Example
Ideas from external sources	Direct suggestions from other individuals, inside of healthcare or as external influencers, may lead to the identification of a researchable problem. Such a problem could have been raised at an institutional research ethics committee.	A healthcare professional could explore the teaching practices of health sciences educators about the teaching strategies used to teach ethical considerations.

Considerations regarding research problems

The researcher should consider the following factors when deciding on the **appropriateness** of a research problem:

- the significance of the study for the health sciences field and for the community
- the originality of the problem
- the benefits of the study
- the researchability of the problem
- the study's feasibility
- the meaningful contribution of the study to evidence-based practice
- the ethical implications of the study.

The study's **significance** is based on the problem identified. Ideally, the research should contribute to society and to health sciences knowledge in a meaningful way. The researcher thus needs to answer the following questions:

- Is the problem an important issue for the discipline?
- Why is the research worth conducting?
- Will patients, healthcare professionals or communities benefit from the study's findings?
- Will the body of knowledge within the field be increased as a result of this study?
- Could the findings aid improvements in healthcare practices or policies?
- Would implementing the study's findings be cost-effective?

If the answer to most of these questions is 'yes', the problem is probably worth pursuing. If the answer to most of the questions is 'no', the researcher should revise or discard the problem. If the answers do not direct the researcher into a definite decision, more work needs to be done on the identification of the problem in order to make a final decision.

The problem's **researchability** is a crucial factor. Not all questions lend themselves to scientific investigation. Value-orientated, or 'should' questions, may require philosophical analysis. Examples include:

- Should heart transplants be performed in provincial hospitals?

- Should abortions in all age groups be permitted?
- Should assisted death as a 'death with dignity' concept be legalised?
- Should additional clinical experience be included in the psychology curriculum requirements?
- What should the home-based caregiver's role be in caring for terminally ill patients?

Value-orientated questions can, however, be revised to focus on beliefs and perceptions of a study's participants or on the impact of the proposed action. For example, the question: 'Should heart transplants be performed in provincial hospitals?' can be changed to: 'How favourably does the community view the moratorium on heart transplants due to financial constraints?'

Research questions that can be answered by a simple 'yes' or 'no' should not be pursued. Examples include:

- Are most academics in South Africa also seasoned researchers?
- Is the frequency of administering pain medication during the night strictly according to doctor's prescription?

Although data can be collected to answer these questions, they do not relate to broader theoretical problems that would encourage the researcher to offer explanations or make predictions. To qualify as 'researchable', the questions must be altered to suggest a reason for data collection. For example, 'Is the frequency of administering pain medication during the night strictly according to a doctor's prescription?' can be restated as: 'What are the prescribed pain medication practices during the night?'

A researchable question is one that yields facts to solve a problem, generates new research, adds to existing theory or improves healthcare practices. It will elicit answers that explain, describe, identify, substantiate, predict or qualify.

Feasibility refers to whether a study can be carried out. Many potentially interesting and useful studies must be discarded because they are not feasible. Factors that may affect the feasibility are time, the researcher's experience, availability of study participants, co-operation of other role players and stakeholders, ethical considerations, facilities and equipment, and funding. To assess feasibility, the researcher must answer the following questions:

- Can this research be completed within the stated timeframe?
- Has adequate provision been made for resources like funding, equipment and access to facilities?
- Will participating in the study have a cost for the participants?
- How easily can research participants be recruited and will they be willing to participate in the study?
- Will I be given permission to carry out the study, and will I gain access to the study field and potential participants? Who would the gatekeepers be?

- Will I be able to reach the research site? Will the study participants be able to travel to the research site?
- Will I be able to obtain approval from the relevant authorities?
- Do I have the expertise to undertake this study?
- Am I sufficiently interested in the research question?

Time is an important factor in the evaluation of a research problem. A novice researcher may have difficulty in estimating how much work is involved and how long the study will take, but the research process steps discussed in Chapter 4 offer a good starting point. Each step should be broken down and time allocated appropriately. A novice should seek the advice of more experienced researchers. Valuable information about locating and accessing resources can also be obtained from librarians and funders.

A study may be delayed for a considerable length of time if permission from authorities and committees is required, and the researcher must take this into consideration. Even well-planned research can take longer than expected or planned, but the total time required should be calculated carefully. For example, if you are required to conduct a research project for an Honours study within six months and you calculate that it will take you a year to complete, your study will not be feasible. You will have to refine it to 'fit' the time limit. Similarly, if you expect to complete a study in a year, but the data collection takes longer, you will need to adapt the research plan.

Working as part of an international research team could be more time-consuming, not only because of the scope of the study, but also because of the time spent on communication, planning, analysis and interpretation of multiple data sets.

Another factor to consider is **resource requirements**, which can vary considerably from one study to another. When undertaking research as part of an Honours course, a study may need minimal resources, while a much more sustained project could require vast quantities of materials (such as copies of instruments), equipment (such as laboratory time and instruments), computers, telecommunication facilities, internet data and so on. A study's design will also influence the number of resources required. Costs incurred as part of literature searches, telephone/internet communication, statistical consultations, language and technical support for report writing, as well as of items such as data, postage, computer access, specialised equipment, travel and office space rental must all be ascertained (these estimates will allow for the feasibility of the study to be accurately assessed). The researcher should also consider whether they have the financial resources required, and whether the anticipated costs outweigh the value of the study's findings. It is unethical for a researcher to embark on a study that they might not be able to complete and to misuse research funds.

In any study involving human participants **participant availability** is an important factor. The researcher needs to decide whether enough people with the desired characteristics will be available and should recognise that potential participants may not be enthusiastic: some may refuse to participate, while others may be reluctant or withdraw.

Another criterion used by reviewers of a research problem is **researcher expertise**. Novice researchers need to understand the concepts and practical skills relevant to conducting research. For example, training in performing focus group interviews is required when researchers are inexperienced.

Motivation is perhaps the most significant prerequisite for undertaking any type of research. Motivation and enthusiasm are indicative of the ability to persist with a task. Even if it entails a relatively simple project, research is a process and requires considerable thought and organisation.

The identified problem does not exist in a vacuum: it is embedded in a particular **context**, and the researcher views it from their philosophical perspective. This means that the researcher's beliefs and values reflect their assumptions, which in turn influence the way they perceive human beings, the environment, health and healthcare.

The researcher's **theoretical and methodological** beliefs about the nature and structure of the problem are preferences, assumptions and presuppositions about what ought to constitute good research. Decisions about how to pursue the problem will be guided by these beliefs and will also define the boundaries and directions of the project.

Research must be ethical, and the researcher is responsible for considering whether their study will meet the criteria for ethical research during all phases of the process.

Formulating a research problem

When formulating the research problem the researcher clarifies what the purpose of the study is for both themselves and others. Subsequent elaboration of method should be oriented to providing information to address that problem. To qualify as a research problem the following are important:

- The problem statement should be clear and concise.
- The problem should relate to one or more fields of study.
- The research problem should be feasible, researchable and significant.
- The research problem should be grounded in theory.
- The research problem must have a base in the literature.

The research problem should consist of the following elements:

- To answer the question 'Why is there a need for this study, investigation or inquiry?' The aim of the problem which is to be investigated must thus be clear.
- To answer the question 'What will be investigated?' The topic or phenomenon which is to be investigated must be clear.

- To answer the question 'When will the study be conducted?' The time dimension in which the study will be conducted is important here.
- To answer the question 'Where will the study be conducted?' The research setting and site must be clear.
- To answer the question 'Who will be the study participants from whom the data will be collected?' This may include individuals, groups, communities and institutions.

Taking into consideration the above, the researcher should follow these guidelines when formulating a research problem:
- Provide enough information to explain what is known and what is not.
- Clearly identify the gap or discrepancy.
- After providing a general discussion of the problem, formulate the problem as a short statement.
- The problem statement could be in either a declarative (statement) or an interrogative (question) form.

A problem must be well-presented and formulated because it serves as the framework from which the study is conceptualised. The problem must be broad enough to explain the researcher's motivation for conducting the study, and also specific enough to provide the research process with direction. The research question, purpose, aim and study objectives are all derived from the problem statement. The research problem thus addresses the 'what' and 'why', whereas the study's purpose addresses the intent. Houser (2008) points out that neither is enough to guide the study design and methods. Therefore, a focused research question or purpose statement is needed. Polit and Beck (2021) state that the problem statement presents the rationale for the study, the purpose statement summarises the aim or goal of the study, and the research question is the specific query a researcher has in addressing the problem. An example is:
- Research problem: Students have been exposed to online learning as a result of the Covid-19 pandemic and the restrictions on social and other contact. Universities provided support in the form of free data for learning purposes. One of the issues that influenced online learning was connectivity and the availability of internet in certain areas of the country.
- Purpose statement: The purpose of the study is to explore and describe the difficulties that university students experienced with online learning during the Covid-19 pandemic.
- Research question: What are the experiences of university students during the Covid-19 pandemic about online learning?

The congruence between the topic, research problem, purpose statement and research question is important. Researchers often refer to the 'golden thread' that should run through a study.

Summary

In this chapter we focused on the research topic and the research problem. Students were introduced to the concepts and how to select a research problem. Factors that researchers must consider when selecting a research problem were discussed, and how to formulate a research problem was demonstrated through examples.

Exercises

1. Discuss at least five sources which could provide research problems for health sciences' studies.
2. Under which circumstances would a problem constitute an inappropriate subject for scientific research?
3. Distinguish between a 'research problem' and a 'research purpose'.
4. Identify a researchable problem and explain why the problem meets the criteria of a researchable problem.
5. Using the same example as in question 4, answer the questions that will determine whether the research problem adheres to all the elements required in a research problem.

The literature review

Chapter 6

LEARNING OUTCOMES

On completion of this chapter, you should be able to demonstrate your understanding of:

- the reasons a literature review is an essential part of research
- the purpose of a literature review
- the differences between primary and secondary sources
- the steps involved in the review process
- how to locate appropriate references
- what critical review means
- reference management software packages
- the guidelines for writing a literature review
- a framework for evaluating the literature review

Once the researcher identifies the topic and the purpose of their study, they must conduct a systematic **search of the literature** to find out what is known about the topic. The literature search and review is a crucial element of the research process and results in a focused, thorough and well-designed study. A literature review is essential in developing an understanding of a given area, limiting the scope of the study and conveying the relevance of the study.

The literature review is usually done at the outset of the study and is updated or extended during the final phase. It aids the researcher in familiarising themselves with the existing knowledge base. The depth of the initial literature review differs for the different research approaches.

Definitions

The literature consists of all the written sources relevant to the topic of interest. A literature review involves finding, reading, understanding and forming conclusions about the published research and theory, as well as presenting it in an organised manner. Gray, Grove and Sutherland (2017) explain that a literature review is a systematic and explicit approach to identifying, retrieving and bibliographically managing independent studies for the purpose of finding information on a topic, making conclusions, recognising areas for future studies, and developing guidelines for practice. Polit and Beck (2021) refer to the literature review as a critical summary of existing knowledge on a topic, often prepared to contextualise the research problem. Thomas (2019) describes literature reviews as a carefully constructed process to establish what previous research has been carried out in the field of interest and that influences one's research. Literature reviews present comprehensive, critical and unbiased evaluations of what is known in the field of study. Thomas (2019) further states that a well-executed review will identify research opportunities or gaps in the literature and provide logical and well-constructed arguments for exploring these gaps to create new knowledge. Literature reviews are often grouped as follows: traditional or narrative, systematic, meta-analysis and meta-synthesis. This chapter focuses on the traditional literature review. Consult sources specifically focused on the different types of reviews should you wish to gain more in-depth information on the different types of reviews.

Purpose of the literature review

Researchers conduct literature reviews for various reasons:

- To conduct a critical and analytical appraisal of recent scholarly work on the topic: in determining what is already known about the topic, the researcher obtains a comprehensive picture of the current knowledge base.
- To identify the research problem and refine research questions.
- To argue the scope and complexity of the research problem.
- To contextualise the study within the general body of knowledge – this minimises the possibility of duplication and increases the probability of a valuable contribution.
- To obtain clues about the methodology and instruments to use: the researcher learns what approaches and methods have, and have not, been attempted, and what data-collecting instruments exist and work or do not work.
- To refine certain aspects of the study: specifically the problem statement, hypothesis, conceptual framework, design and the data analysis process.
- To compare existing studies' findings with those of the proposed study – this process also demonstrates the relevance of the proposed study to the existing body of knowledge.
- To inform or support a qualitative study, especially in conjunction with data collection and analysis.

The specific aims of the literature review depend on the researcher's role. They can use the review to acquire knowledge, to critique existing practices, to develop research-based protocols and interventions, to develop a theory or conceptual framework, or to develop policy statements, curricula or practice guidelines (Burns & Grove, 2017).

Literature reviews do not necessarily always form part of a planned study, but can be compiled as a stand-alone activity and published as such. Free standing reviews can take on various forms such as narrative literature reviews, systematic reviews, scoping reviews, integrative reviews and more recently mixed-methods literature reviews. An example would be: Effectiveness of e-Health interventions on psychosocial health for infertile patients: a systematic review and meta-analysis (Sigma, 2022).

The purpose of a literature review in **quantitative research** is to direct the study's planning and execution. The main literature review is conducted at the start of the study, while another is done at the end to identify and integrate relevant sources published since the original literature review. The research report contains discussions of both literature reviews, and relevant sources are cited throughout. The introduction contains sources which aided the development of the study's focus. The literature review includes both theoretical and empirical literature which addresses current knowledge of the phenomenon under investigation. The research methods section includes sources which validate the methods selected (such as design, population, sampling, data collection, data analysis and ethical consideration). In the results section the present study's data are compared with the results of existing studies. The last part of the report, containing the discussions, provides a synthesis of findings from existing and present studies.

The purpose and timing of the literature review in **qualitative research** varies according to the type (design) of study conducted. Although the literature is reviewed to some extent to explore the broader topic, and to make the researcher aware of the existing knowledge, the actual literature review is conducted at a later stage than in quantitative studies. In phenomenological studies the literature should be reviewed after data collection and analysis to prevent the researcher's impartiality being compromised. The information from the literature is then compared with the findings of the study to determine current knowledge of a phenomenon. When grounded theory is used, the literature explains, supports and extends the theory generated in the study. Ethnographic researchers, like quantitative researchers, review the literature early on to provide a general understanding and background of the variables explored. Historical research requires an extensive literature review, which consists of an initial review (to develop research questions) and another search and review to develop a source of data which explains a phenomenon over a particular time period.

Mixed methods studies vary in their outline and when to conduct the literature review. All mixed methods studies will include the initial literature review as described above. In exploratory mixed methods design where the study commences with the qualitative phase, an integrative review could be a typical way of exploring the literature. In an explanatory mixed methods design that commences with a quantitative phase, or a concurrent mixed methods design, a systematic or traditional literature review could be one of the first steps in the research process. More detail on mixed methods research should be explored in research sources specifically focusing on mixed methods designs.

Types of information and sources

Polit and Beck (2021) divide the types of information to be included in a literature review into five categories:

1. Facts, statistics and research findings
2. Theories or interpretations
3. Methods and procedures
4. Opinions, beliefs or points of view
5. Anecdotes, clinical impressions or narrations of incidents and situations.

1. Facts, statistics and research findings

This category constitutes one of the most important types of information for a literature review. Research findings suggest topics for investigation and can help the researcher to conceptualise and design new research. It is useful for the researcher to review research findings in health sciences literature as well as in the literature of related disciplines (such as sociology, psychology, anthropology, education and management). A good literature review includes current, relevant literature as well as material of historical interest (if relevant to the phenomenon under investigation). In some instances 'classic' sources (also referred to as 'seminal' studies/sources) add value to research methodology: an example is Lincoln and Guba's (1985) work explaining trustworthiness in qualitative research. Seminal sources refer to older sources that are still relevant and important in current times. They are often described as landmark sources that made a large impact within a particular discipline and continue to be referenced in current research. They typically contained new ideas when published and continue to have an influence in the field within which they are published or to which they are relevant.

2. Theories or interpretations

This category deals with broader, more conceptual issues of relevance. For example, if you wish to research reflective practices in teaching and learning, you would search the literature for various reflective practice theories and models; if you are concerned with the particular needs of certain patients, you would search for theories on patient needs. Descriptions of theories are useful in providing a conceptual context for your research problem, and of course for your research question and study design.

3. Methods and procedures

In this category, the researcher deals with methods of conducting a study. That is, in reviewing the literature, the researcher should pay attention not only to what has been found, but also to how it was found. They should pose the following questions:

- Which approaches were used previously?
- How have other researchers operationalised and measured variables?
- How have study participants been selected and included in the study?
- How have researchers controlled the research situation to enhance interpretation?
- Which statistical methods have been used for data analysis?

4. Opinions, beliefs or points of view

Articles focusing on their authors' opinions are subjective and present suggestions and points of view of one or several individuals. If a study focuses on controversial or 'emerging' issues in the field, so-called 'opinion articles' can be a valuable source of ideas. Articles that are reflective papers may not have all the methodological steps required of a research report, but could add important value to the literature review. These types of articles may stimulate prospective researchers to engage in a project to provide scientific evidence on a particular topic or phenomenon.

5. Anecdotes, clinical impressions or narrations of incidents and situations

This category may serve to broaden the researcher's understanding of a problem, particularly if they are unfamiliar with underlying issues. While these sources may demonstrate a need for rigorous research, they have limited utility in literature reviews for research studies because of their highly subjective nature. The researcher should not rely on them in their review of the literature, but if they decide to include them, they should be supplemented with scientific sources.

The sources can be categorised as either theoretical or empirical. **Theoretical sources** include concept analyses, theories, models and conceptual frameworks. They can be found in periodicals, monographs and conference proceedings, but also in journal articles where they are applied or in research sources where they are provided as examples. **Empirical sources** contain knowledge derived from research and are found in journals and books, and in unpublished formats such as conference proceedings and theses.

Primary and secondary sources

Primary sources are those reports written by the person who originated or is responsible for generating the ideas or data. There are two broad types of **primary sources:** research studies and statistical reports. Research studies range in scope from small pilot studies to broad-based, controlled experiments – and thus refer to empirical sources. In the health sciences primary sources include diaries, letters, interviews, eyewitness accounts, speeches, documents and autobiographies. A **primary theoretical source** is written by a theorist who has developed a specific theory or concept.

Secondary sources summarise or quote content from primary sources, thus paraphrasing the work of other researchers and theorists. While useful, these sources rely on an author's interpretation of someone else's work, which may result in the source being shaped and influenced by the author's perceptions and biases. Indeed, errors and misrepresentation of facts have been promulgated in some instances. The researcher should strive to locate and utilise primary sources when undertaking a study whenever possible, because they provide the least biased evidence.

Depth and breadth of the review

The **depth** of a literature review refers to the number and quality of sources the researcher examines, while the **breadth** is determined by the variety. If the literature review is too broad, the researcher may have included inapplicable sources, and if it lacks sufficient depth and breadth, they may have overlooked important ones. The literature review's depth and breadth depend on the researcher's background, the complexity of the research topic and the amount of relevant literature available. The depth of a review is also enhanced by a critical assessment of the study's methodological quality.

Developing a search strategy

The literature search should be based on wide-ranging interpretations of the research topic. By keeping the research topic and question in mind when conducting the initial search, reading the materials, and identifying keywords and concepts in the title of the study, the researcher hones the focus of the searches, and thus increases the rigour of the review. The purpose of the literature review should also be kept in mind. Therefore, selecting keywords and concepts relevant to a study entails a process of analysing the topic, title, purpose of the literature review and relevant variables. As relevant sources are identified and explored, these can serve as further information for more relevant keywords.

To identify search terms and their correct spellings, the researcher may scan titles and abstracts for relevance. In doing so, they are acquainted with topics in the field, what key words are used and who the prominent researchers are. Criteria which help to focus the search are the date of publication, period of interest, language preference and exclusion, databases to use, types of studies and exclusion criteria.

Using libraries and electronic databases

Recently literature searches are mainly done through electronic databases. However, some researchers still use libraries in addition to electronic databases as their sources of their research literature. Most libraries have inter-library loan services and access to electronic databases. Databases give researchers access to a wide variety of sources.

Researchers should acquaint themselves with a library's facilities and staff. Librarians can assist with indexes, reference materials and computer-assisted searches: indeed, often the most complex part of a literature search is identifying the material, not obtaining it. Although hand searches are limited to libraries, this method gives the researcher access to sources which may not be indexed on electronic databases.

Electronic data searches require a computer, access to the internet and a systematic plan that includes a clear research question or purpose as well as keywords or concepts. The assistance of a librarian can be valuable, especially to a novice researcher. Multiple databases should be considered, as all available sources will not necessarily appear on a specific database. The search must be specific about identifying relevant sources as extensively as possible.

Identifying sources

In conducting an in-depth search of the literature, the researcher must first clarify the research topic, identify keywords and concepts, and then identify all relevant publications in the area of interest. (Using Boolean logic to frame the database search is very helpful. A Boolean search uses key words connected by the logical operators 'and', 'or', 'with', 'not'.) By using a combination of keywords and one or more of the Boolean operators, one could narrow down the search and focus on the specific area of interest (Machi & McEvoy, 2016).

'Relevance' refers to how closely information relates to the topic. For example, a researcher interested in studying the relationship between obesity and dietary patterns in teenagers would try to find research which:

- examines this question
- examines related questions (for example, eating patterns of successful dieters, factors influencing obesity, diets in obesity and the general eating patterns of teenagers)
- relates to the concepts of obesity, teenagers and dietary patterns
- relates to the characteristics of obese teenagers.

There are several basic types of search resources:

- Indexes covering various fields of study, and which are used to find journal or periodical references. Examples include the International Nursing Index (INI), the Cumulative Index to Nursing and Allied Health Literature (CINAHL) and Index Medicus.
- Books and journals databases available at libraries. Generally, the catalogue contains an alphabetical listing of books into categories like title, author and subject heading.
- Abstracts, which comprise brief summaries of articles (Dissertation Abstracts International (DAI) is a comprehensive source of doctoral dissertation abstracts in North America).
- Electronic literature searches. There are many useful electronic databases for research, including the following:
  - Nursing and Allied Health. Various databases such as ProQuest, EBSCOhost, Sabinet, AJOL and more provide access to this database.
  - Medline. This database corresponds to three printed indexes: Index Medicus, INI and the Index to Dental Literature.
  - Search engines such as Google Scholar, Pubmed, Cochrane, CDC and Medscape.
  - Librarians can assist in identifying relevant indexes or search engines.
- Local resources. These include the completed research lists of the Human Sciences Research Council (HSRC), the Medical Research Council (MRC), the National Research Foundation (NRF) and other professional bodies.
- The Union Catalogue of Theses and Dissertations (UCTD) contains bibliographic information about theses and dissertations submitted to South African universities (at Master's and doctoral level).

In electronic searches, keywords and phrases are entered into a computer program or internet browser, and a list of relevant articles returned. Researchers should make use of the assistance of a librarian when using these resources. Novice researchers should invest in a 'critical friend' or research mentor to assist and support them in this process. When conducting collaborative research, co-researchers are important for support with the specific searching of sources. The reference list which appears at the end of every article is a useful means of finding other relevant literature.

Locating sources

To locate sources, the researcher must follow these steps:

- compile a list of identified sources
- search for them
- systematically record the references
- determine additional means of locating sources.

Compiling lists of identified sources and searching for them

The researcher can compile their list of sources in several ways. One could sort sources according to topics, keywords or themes by creating categories for each of the specific topics. Journal sources can be organised according to journal name and year of publication. For example, if most of the sources are from the *Journal of Advanced Nursing, Nursing Research,* the *Journal of Nursing Education* and the *International Nursing Review*, the researcher could group the articles from each together and organise them according to the year of publication. This prevents the researcher from simply wandering from one journal to the next.

Various reference management software programs exist such as Mendeley, OneNote, EndNote, X9, Zotero and Citavi. Not all are free software packages, but they are none the less very helpful in organising one's sources. The software package allows researchers to collect, organise and use bibliographic references or citations. The text citations can be transferred from the bibliography to the text, making it much easier to reference correctly. The package also allows the researcher to make notes on and highlight sections in the articles that appear on the personal profile of the researcher. Although we live in an electronic era, it is often useful to print out electronic sources to make the processes of reading them and writing up the literature review easier. A systematic filing system ordered according to author name or key concepts allows the researcher to easily locate printed sources.

The review process

The process of reviewing literature has changed considerably. Access to computers and international electronic databases enables researchers to find and retrieve relevant sources quickly. In reviewing literature, the researcher should:

- locate sources
- read sources critically
- make notes and highlight where relevant
- write the review report
- evaluate the review report.

Systematically recording references

The researcher must establish a systematic method for recording information. They can enter and save information into their personal profile on the reference management system, an electronic folder or file, or via a manual, handwritten system. Whatever the method selected, the sources should be filed alphabetically according to author or title. Categories can then be created according to topics, authors, journals or year of publication.

Each entry should include:
- the name(s) of the author(s)
- the date of publication
- the title of the article, report or book
- the name of the journal or publisher
- the volume and number of the journal
- the place of publication (in the case of a book)
- relevant page numbers
- the researcher's notes.

The notes the researcher makes will be determined by the reason why the source was selected and could contain:
- the problem statement
- the definition of concepts
- hypotheses (if any)
- theories or assumptions used
- research method (if applicable)
- instruments used (if applicable)
- data analysis method (if applicable)
- findings and summaries
- recommendations of importance to the researcher
- the researcher's evaluation of each of these aspects.

Careful note-taking and reference citation facilitate the rest of the research process. A systematic recording process increases the accuracy and completeness of the reference list or bibliography. Software such as EndNote and Mendeley's Reference Manager can also be used to organise references and are very helpful in presenting the sources in the required reference style.

Determining additional ways of locating sources

Even the largest libraries do not contain every text for which the researcher may have a relevant reference. Similarly, electronic searches do not always reveal these sought-after sources either. The researcher may need to use services such as inter-library loans (which can be time-consuming). For historical or ethnographic studies artefacts and other cultural sources may be found elsewhere.

Reading sources critically

Reading critically involves a preliminary phase and a critical review. In the **preliminary phase** the researcher reads the abstract and scans the article, chapter or report in order to determine whether it is suitable for review. They then critically review the relevant sections, which entails analysing the usability, completeness and consistency of the piece, evaluating its strengths and weaknesses, and assessing its relevance in relation to their own study. The **critical review** helps the researcher evaluate every decision taken in each step of the research process. It therefore involves questioning assumptions and claims made for which no evidence has been provided, considering the findings of one researcher compared to another, and then evaluating them.

Writing the review report

When composing the literature review, the researcher studies the literature in detail, but does not report on the whole literature review. It is not appropriate for the researcher to try to include everything, and they should rather report on the portions which are relevant and directly related to the study's problem and purpose. It is essential that the review is scientifically adequate or clinically applicable.

The literature review must have a clear structure and logical flow. Machi and McEvoy (2016) provide an example of a typical literature review outline:

- Introduction section of the literature review
  - Introductory statement
  - Study topic statement
  - Context statement
  - Significance statement
  - Problem statement
  - Organisation statement
- Body section of the literature review
  - Discovery argument: Background section presenting a current understanding of the topic
  - Advocacy argument: Conclusions section presenting findings and conclusions that argue the claim (research question)
- Summary of the literature review
  - Answer the research question
  - Conclude the analysis
  - Study implications.

The researcher must therefore pay attention to the following:

- The literature review must present a thoughtful analysis and synthesis of the literature and should not merely comprise a collection of quotations and conclusions. Simply gathering quotations from various sources fails to show whether existing research has been assimilated and understood.
- The literature review should begin with an introduction which should refer to the sources consulted and give an indication of the body of work currently in existence. The introduction should also briefly describe the review's structure and purpose in order to guide the reader and contextualise the elements.
- The body of the review should consist of a critique of existing work, as well as a theoretical dimension. The researcher should begin by describing the literature on the independent variable and then discuss the dependent variable(s) and their relationships.
- Source content should be paraphrased or summarised and should reveal the current state of knowledge on the subject.
- Direct quotations may be used to emphasise central issues. If they are, they should be as short as possible – long quotations are often unnecessary and tend to interfere with the reader's train of thought. Quotations should be reproduced exactly, and they should not be used out of context, as the significance may be lost, or the reader may misinterpret them. A reference used in-text for a quotation must include the page number of the quotation.
- Full credit must be given to the author(s) of the original work. If this is not done, the researcher is guilty of plagiarism and could be liable for prosecution. Author(s) are credited in-text by having their name(s) and the year of publication indicated, and in some reference styles, the page numbers. Moreover, full details of author(s), publication date(s), title, publisher and place of publication must be provided in a reference list at the end of the chapter or text. There are different systems according to which the reference list may be compiled: for example, the Harvard system, the adapted Harvard system, APA and the Vancouver system. None of these is necessarily more 'correct' than the other, but whatever system is selected, it must be applied consistently.
- The review should be as objective as possible. A text which fails to support the researcher's hypothesis or that conflicts with their personal values should not be omitted. Material obtained from sources should not be distorted to support the selected problem.
- The review should be balanced: it should identify the strengths and weaknesses of each reference and should compare differences and similarities between them. In other words, the review must reflect every aspect of the issue.
- The review should include the most up-to-date information. Recent sources are often described as sources not older than five years, but this may differ from institution to institution, researcher to researcher, topic to topic. Good practice, however, is to include sources not older than ten years or justify the reasons for using older sources. For example, where a topic is researched that is trendy, such as online learning or the effect of lockdown regulations on the mental health of the community, one would use recent sources given the topical nature of the phenomenon under study.

- The review should conclude with a summary of synthesised findings of existing work. The summary should also point out gaps in the literature, or areas of 'research inactivity'.

Evaluating the research review

Researchers must evaluate not only the literature they review, but also their own interpretations. Pertinent questions include the following:

- Is the review comprehensive?
- Is it relevant to the problem at hand?
- Is it up to date?
- Are all aspects of the issue presented?
- Is there sound research-based evidence?
- Are secondary sources used excessively?
- Does it critically appraise the contribution of key studies?
- Is it organised logically?
- Is it sufficiently objective?

Summary

In this chapter we explained that the main functions of a literature review are to provide an up-to-date account of what is known about the study topic, to provide a conceptual and theoretical context, to assist the researcher in obtaining clues to the methodology and instrumentation, and to refine certain parts of the study. We pointed out that the type of information to be included in the review is divided into five broad categories, and that literature sources are classified as either primary or secondary. We discussed in detail the five steps or components of the review process, in which we proposed that the review should present a thoughtful analysis of the field and not simply a collection of quotations and summaries. An outline of how the review report could be presented was provided. Furthermore, it should include all published points of view rather than simply those that support the researcher's view. Finally, we pointed out that the literature review must be submitted to the same critical analysis and ethical assessment as is the rest of the research process.

Exercises

1. Select an article from a health sciences journal and evaluate its literature review.

2. Comment on the following aspects of the research article selected in question 1:

   (a) the relevance of the literature to the problem

   (b) the use of primary sources and secondary sources

   (c) the current nature of the literature

   (d) the use of empirical material versus theory and opinion.

3. You want to investigate the needs of healthcare professionals working in critical care units for emotional support. List the key concepts and phrases that would aid your literature search.

4. Search for an article on communication skills in the healthcare environment. Use the bibliography of the article to search for five more recent articles and justify your choice in terms of the data of publication.

5. Select any ten sources from this textbook's bibliography. Indicate which of these are primary sources and which are secondary sources.

6. Choose any of the reference manager software packages that are freely available. Create a site and capture ten articles on your personal profile. The articles must cover three different topics to allow you to create three categories in your profile.

Refining and defining the research question

Once the researcher identifies a researchable problem, a clear question is formulated, and the research aims and objectives are determined. The conceptualisation process may take time and requires creative thinking. The nature of the research question determines the study design, data sources and sampling strategies, data collection, analysis and interpretation. A fundamental factor is addressing the research question in a systematic, rigorous and ethical way. This chapter covers how to formulate a clear research question.

Refining the research question

The research question narrows down a broad topic to a focused area that is addressed in a study. When formulating research questions, it is important to distinguish between questions that can be answered through research and those for which research will not elicit answers. If the research problem is complex, the research question often entails one or more questions. For example, a researcher working in a clinic has identified a high rate of unplanned teenage pregnancies as an area of concern. Questions that may arise include:

- What sexual behaviours do teenagers engage in?
- How effective is the health education programme on sexual health provided to teenagers?

Several specific research questions such as the following could result:
- What sexual behaviours do teenagers engage in?
- What is the correlation between the rate of pregnancy among teenage girls and health education on sexual health?
- How effective is the health education programme on sexual health?
- How do pregnant teenagers experience the unplanned pregnancy?

Although these questions have a similar theme, each is unique and can be studied using different approaches. Each has a specific focus, is clearly articulated and can give the study direction, because they have been transformed into a manageable, researchable question.

Reformulating a research problem in question form helps the researcher to delineate the problem. Once a clear research question is formulated, the researcher can establish the study's purpose. A purpose statement should include:
- the research aim (specified with terms such as 'to identify', 'to describe', 'to explore', 'to explain' and 'to predict')
- the target population
- the setting
- the research variables.

For example, 'The purpose of this study is to describe the unplanned pregnancies among teenagers in the Mahapani community'. The aim here is to 'describe', the target population is 'pregnant teenagers', the setting is 'Mahapani community' and the research variable is 'sexual behaviour'. In this case only a single variable is described. If the purpose of the study is to determine the efficacy of the health education programme on the incidence of pregnancies in teenagers residing in Mahapani community, two variables would have to be considered: sexual behaviour and teenage pregnancy.

Once the research question and purpose are formulated, the researcher needs to determine whether the area of concern has been properly addressed. They can do this by posing the following questions:
- Does the problem statement address the area of concern clearly and concisely?
- Is the purpose clearly formulated?
- How feasible is it to study the problem and purpose?
- Does the purpose clarify or limit the focus or aims of the study?
- Will the question(s) and purpose generate knowledge for the field?
- Will the purpose of the study be ethical?

- Am I experienced enough to conduct the study?
- Will the study's findings have an impact on healthcare?

Research questions and hypotheses, as well as the aims and objectives of a study, result from the more abstractly stated research problem and purpose (once these have been examined for significance and feasibility). The aim and objectives are formulated to bridge the gap between the problem, purpose and the detailed design and plan for data collection and analysis, while some theorists differentiate only between questions and/or hypotheses, and the aims and objectives.

Research questions

Example 7.1 demonstrates how a research purpose is refined into a research question using the interrogative form. The study centres on the portrayal of nurses' knowledge in research reports in medical and other health-related journals.

Example 7.1

The purpose of the study is to examine the content of articles in medical and health-related journals in order to determine if the reporting of nurses' knowledge reflects their academic qualifications.

The study addresses the following questions:
- What reports of nurses' knowledge are described in articles appearing in medical and other health-related journals?
- How do these reports differ from the actual knowledge nurses display in practising in the healthcare system?
- To what extent is the reporting of nurses stereotypical, particularly about nurses' knowledge levels and qualifications?

Research questions narrow a study's focus. Those formulated for qualitative studies tend to be more general in emphasis and include concepts which are more complex and abstract than those typically found in quantitative studies.

Example 7.2 demonstrates research questions formulated for a qualitative study.

Example 7.2

The purpose of the study is to explore the characteristics of women who successfully manage their weight.

The following questions are addressed:
- What weight management methods are used by women who successfully manage their weight?
- What factors influence the selection of particular methods?

Thus, Examples 7.1 and 7.2 show that the research problem, purpose, questions and objectives need to be clear, logical and focused, as well as showing how they direct the remaining steps of the research process.

Babbie and Mouton (2021) mention two broad categories of questions – empirical and non-empirical questions. Empirical questions are formulated to answer what can be measured and observed. Non-empirical questions are used for research that is interpretive in nature, often involving processes and aspects that cannot be observed directly (Du Plooy-Cilliers et al, 2014).

Examples of empirical questions are:

- Exploratory questions: questions that address the 'what?' questions, such as 'What are the factors affecting non-disclosure of HIV status to a sexual partner?'
- Descriptive questions: questions that address the 'how?' questions, such as 'How does body mass index affect the recovery of a patient after surgery?'
- Causal questions: questions that address the 'why?' questions, such as 'Why does music therapy result in lower blood pressure in elderly patients?'
- Evaluative questions: questions that address the outcome or success of an initiative, such as 'How has the implementation of the mother-and-baby-friendly initiative improved exclusive breastfeeding?'
- Predictive questions: questions that address the effect of one aspect of a situation on another, such as 'What effect do the rules and regulations of a medical aid have on the choice of doctor?'
- Historical questions: questions that address the investigation of history, historical events or how these events influence the current situation, such as 'How do the professional organisations influence the training of nurses in South Africa?'

Examples of non-empirical questions are:

- Conceptual questions: questions that attempt to determine the meaning of a construct, such as 'What is cultural competent care?'
- Theoretical questions: questions that attempt to identify appropriate theories, models and conceptual frameworks, such as 'What is the theoretical underpinning of the Watson's Theory of Human Caring?'
- Meta-analytical questions: questions that attempt to determine the current debates and trends regarding a particular topic, such as 'How is mindfulness integrated into caring science theory?'
- Normative or philosophical questions: questions that address issues of an ideal state of being, such as 'What constitutes the ideal nurse?'

Research hypotheses

A hypothesis is a set of assumptions about observable phenomena that are expressed in a coherent manner. It is the formal statement comprising a researcher's prediction or explanation of the relationship between two or more variables in a specific population. In other words, the hypothesis translates the problem statement into a prediction of expected outcomes, based on theoretical considerations. The hypothesis is therefore a statement that the researchers will attempt to accept or reject when examining the results at the end of a study.

In quantitative research, hypotheses are typically used to direct correlational, quasi-experimental or experimental studies and to test theories. Research methodology hypotheses for healthcare professionals sometimes follow directly from a theoretical framework. Hypotheses must be tested empirically before they can be accepted and incorporated into a theory. If a hypothesis is not supported by empirical evidence, it must be rejected, and the researcher is obliged to suggest another hypothesis. The role of the hypothesis is thus not only to make predictions or to explain certain facts or problems, but also to guide the investigation and provide focus for the study.

When a researcher is testing a hypothesis, they are not trying to 'prove' it to be true. Rather, the researcher wants to find out whether there is one case that will falsify the hypothesis. If one is unable to find such a case, the only thing that one can 'prove' is that one cannot 'disprove' the hypothesis. Therefore, the more supporting evidence there is for the hypothesis, the higher the probability that it is correct, resulting in the ability to make predictions and formulate theories (Du Plooy-Cilliers et al, 2014).

The main characteristics of operational hypotheses include:

- A statement of the predicted relationship between two or more variables. For example, the statement 'Persons with hypercholesterolemia who have greater knowledge of their disease will have a higher rate of adherence to the treatment regimen than persons with lesser knowledge' suggests a predicted relationship between knowledge and adherence to the treatment regimen. Knowledgeable persons will have a higher rate of adherence, whilst those with little knowledge will have a lower rate. This can be regarded as a workable hypothesis as it contains two concepts – adherence and knowledge – that are likely to vary.
- Let us consider whether the following statement relates to workable research: 'Persons with hypercholesterolemia who follow a structured programme have a high rate of adherence to the treatment regimen.' This statement expresses no anticipated relationship as there is only one variable – the person's adherence to treatment. If a statement lacks phrases such as 'more than', 'less than', 'different from' or 'related to', it is not amenable to scientific testing because there is no criterion for assessing absolute outcomes and cannot be called a 'hypothesis'.
- Hypotheses must be conceptually clear and specific and should be stated as simply as possible. All identified variables must be described using operational definitions.
- A hypothesis should be consistent with an existing body of research findings and with logical reasoning. It must not predict results that are inherently contradictory.
- A hypothesis must be testable.
- A hypothesis must relate to a matter that can be clearly defined empirically.

Types of hypotheses

The type of hypothesis formulated is determined by the study's purpose. Common hypothetical classifications include: directional versus non-directional, simple versus complex and null versus research.

A directional hypothesis predicts an outcome in a specific direction. For example, 'Patients with hypercholesterolemia who have followed a structured programme on their condition will be more compliant than those who have not.' In this example, the phrase 'more compliant than' indicates the direction of the hypothesis. Phrases such as 'greater than', 'smaller than', 'more than', 'less than', 'positively' and 'negatively' all indicate direction.

The non-directional hypothesis indicates that a difference or correlation exists, but does not specify an anticipated direction. For example, 'There is a correlation between the satisfaction with remuneration packages reported by South African healthcare professionals and their desire to seek employment in other countries.'

The directional hypothesis is preferred for a health sciences research study if previous studies have demonstrated contradictory findings.

A simple hypothesis (sometimes referred to as 'bivariate') contains only two variables: an independent variable and a dependent variable. The mathematical representation of a simple associative hypothesis (in which variables X and Y are related to, or associated with, one another) is demonstrated in Figure 7.1:

$$X \updownarrow Y$$

Figure 7.1 The mathematical representation of a simple associative hypothesis

The mathematical representation of a simple causal hypothesis in which X is the cause of Y is demonstrated in Figure 7.2:

$$X \longrightarrow Y$$

Figure 7.2 The mathematical representation of a simple causal hypothesis

The following are examples of simple hypotheses:

- There is a direct relationship between income and malnutrition.
- Health education influences the adherence to wound care practices of mothers whose babies have had surgery.

A complex hypothesis (sometimes referred to as 'multivariate') predicts relationships between three or more variables. There may be two or more independent variables, and one or more dependent variables, or vice versa.

The mathematical expression of a complex causal hypothesis with two independent variables – X1 and X2 – and one dependent variable Y, is demonstrated in Figure 7.3:

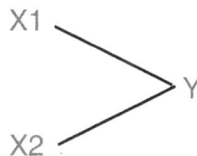

Figure 7.3 The mathematical expression of a complex causal hypothesis with two independent variables and one dependent variable

Examples of complex hypotheses include:

- Daily weight loss is greater for adults who follow a calorie-reduced diet and exercise daily than for those who do not.
- Persons who participate in daily wellness programmes have lower stress levels, higher physical functioning and fewer adverse symptoms than those who do not.

The researcher should be cautious when using complex hypotheses as they can be difficult to measure. In some instances a complex hypothesis can be broken down into simple hypotheses. The null hypothesis (also referred to as a 'statistical' hypothesis) is used for statistical testing and interpreting statistical outcomes. It states that no difference exists between groups, or that there is no correlation between variables, for example, 'There is no relationship between mental health issues and nationality.' If there is no statistically significant difference between nationalities, the null hypothesis is supported, but if a difference in mental health issues between people from different nationalities exists, the null hypothesis is rejected.

In terms of hypothesis testing, the two most important variables are dependent and independent variables. A research hypothesis states that a difference, or correlation, between two or more variables exists. All hypotheses given above are research hypotheses.

Formulating hypotheses

Formulating a hypothesis does not have specific rules, but you should be guided by the following:

Ensure that the hypothesis

- is related to the research question
- assists in solving the research problem
- assists in achieving the aim of the study.

The following aspects must be considered:

- Identify the idea or theory you would like to test by basing the hypothesis on the literature, theory, model or conceptual framework chosen for the study.
- Have a clear purpose for the study and know what you want to achieve.
- Identify the dependent and independent variables.
- The relationship between the variables must relate to specific words such as 'a comparison between', 'greater than', 'differs from', 'a positive correlation between', 'if … then'.
- State the independent variable first, followed by the dependent variable.

A researcher can ask the following questions when refining the hypothesis:

- Is the hypothesis based on the research problem?
- Is the hypothesis logically linked to the research question?
- Is the hypothesis testable?
- Does the hypothesis include the independent and dependent variables?
- Is it possible that the hypothesis can be fabricated?

Research aims and objectives

The aim and objectives are concrete, measurable ends towards which research is directed. Where a study's aim is less specific, the research objectives are defined as clear, concise, declarative statements articulated in the present tense. You will find some authors using these terms synonymously, but we differentiate between them in specificity. An objective usually focuses on one or two variables, and indicates whether they are to be identified, analysed or described. Sometimes, an objective's focus includes identifying relationships between variables and determining differences between two groups using selected variables. The research objectives formulated for qualitative and quantitative studies have similarities because they focus on exploration, description and determining relationships. Because research objectives in qualitative studies focus on obtaining a holistic, comprehensive understanding of the area of study, they are usually broader in focus and include more abstract and complex concepts than those in quantitative studies.

Researchers may state objectives in cases where little (or no) research on a problem exists, and where the study's purpose is to identify or describe characteristics of variables, or to identify relationships between them. For example, a study conducted on the magnitude of lower back problems in healthcare professionals demonstrates the flow of logic from research problem and purpose to conducting the research.

Example 7.3

The purpose of the study is to describe the prevalence and nature of lower back problems in healthcare professionals. The objectives are:

- to determine the prevalence of lower back problems in healthcare professionals

- to ascertain differences between healthcare professionals with occupational back problems and those without in relation to age, work experience and perceived number of lifting patients per shift
- to determine the amount of work time lost, the change in daily activities, the perceived precipitating factors (if any) and the setting in which the lower back problems occur
- to determine whether healthcare professionals have considered leaving the profession because of back pain and problems.

This example illustrates that the study's objectives derive from the research problem and purpose, and that they refine the problem and purpose to provide greater detail on precisely what the researcher is going to examine.

Identifying variables

Variables are the qualities, properties or characteristics of persons, things or situations that change or vary. A variable can therefore take on more than one possible value. For example, the variable 'gender' may take the values of male and female. 'Age' can express many more values, such as under 20 years, 21–30 years or 80–100+. Variables such as 'academic success', 'stress', 'pain' and 'satisfaction' can all take on more than two values.

Types of variables

Since a variable is a quantifiable element which changes or varies, the researcher may have to manage and assess several of them. Some variables can be manipulated, whilst others can be controlled. Some are identified, but not measured, whilst others are measured with refined measurement devices.

Independent variables

Also known as a 'treatment' or 'experimental' variable, the independent variable influences others, and is thus an agent for change. It is perceived as contributing to, or preceding, a particular outcome. In experiments the researcher manipulates the independent variable and performs interventions or treatments to view the resulting change on the dependent variable.

Dependent variables

The dependent variable is the 'outcome' variable, as it reflects the effect of, or response to, the independent variable. It is the variable that appears, disappears, diminishes or amplifies – or changes – as the experiment introduces, removes or varies the independent variable. One example is a study which attempts to demonstrate the effects of an exercise programme on patients with occlusions of the major leg arteries. The dependent variables include the distance walked by the patient to the limit of pain tolerance. The independent variable is the exercise programme, which includes daily walking with the intention of increasing the distance regularly. In a study to determine the effects of salt intake on hypertension, blood pressure is the dependent variable, while salt intake is the independent variable.

There is nothing about a variable which makes it independent or dependent: the use of the variable in a problem under investigation is the defining factor. For example, in a study to determine the effect of health education on post-operative anxiety, 'anxiety' is the dependent variable, while 'giving or withholding health education' is the independent variable. By contrast, in a study to determine the effects of anxiety on post-surgical pain, 'anxiety' is the independent variable, while 'pain' is the dependent variable.

Extraneous variables

These variables are uncontrolled, but nevertheless influence the study's findings. An extraneous variable impacts the independent X and dependent Y variables, giving the impression of a relationship between them, when in fact both X and Y change because of a third variable's variation. In experimental and quasi-experimental research, extraneous variables are areas of concern, and are considered 'threats' to internal and external validity. Examples include the passage of time, mortality, selection bias, instrumentation and maturity.

Extraneous variables are not always recognised and are, by their very nature, uncontrolled. Nevertheless, the researcher should attempt to control them as they may influence the study's outcomes.

Demographic variables

Also called 'attribute variables', demographic variables cannot be manipulated or influenced, but they may be present, and may vary, in the population under study. Examples include research participants' characteristics such as gender, age, race, marital status, religion and educational level. The researcher analyses these variables to form a picture of the sample.

Research variables

Research variables are measurable concepts in studies where a single phenomenon is being examined. They are logical groupings of the phenomenon's attributes, characteristics or traits. Identified in the research purpose, objectives or questions, they are used when the researcher intends to observe or measure variables in their natural states without implementing a treatment. There is no manipulation of an independent variable, nor is there an examination of a cause–effect relationship. An example is a qualitative study which describes patients' experiences of epidural pain relief during labour.

Defining variables

The variables and terms contained in the hypothesis or research question must be clearly defined. Two kinds of definitions are generally required:

1. a conceptual or 'dictionary' definition
2. an operational definition.

Conceptual definitions are more than dictionary (denotative) definitions. They include associated meanings that the word may have. These definitions are described as being connotative, as the terms bring to mind subtle or indirect meanings, feelings or images (Grove et al, 2018). In a conceptual definition a set of concepts defines another concept. For example, a conceptual definition of nurse may include images of a person with a white uniform wearing distinguishing devices, feelings of safety and security, and comfort. The dictionary definition is narrower in that it describes the role of the person in rendering care to others. The definition conveys the theoretical meaning of the concept and describes its properties. Thus, a hungry person could be conceptually defined as someone who needs food, and 'post-operative pain' can be described as the discomfort an individual experiences after surgery.

A conceptual definition is neither true nor false and may or may not be a useful means of communication in a research report. To be useful a conceptual definition should:

- denote distinctive characteristics of what is being defined, for example, the distinctive characteristic of a person in pain is the need for pain medication
- not describe something using the same concepts or terminology, for example, post-operative pain should not be defined as the pain a patient experiences after an operation
- be explicit and clear to avoid ambiguity, for example, defining a substance as a 'drug' presents two interpretations: the substance could be either medicinal or narcotic
- encompass all aspects of the idea the researcher wishes to convey
- be meaningful, and have meaning, within a particular theoretical context
- reflect the theory used in the study
- be appropriate to, and for, the study
- be consistent with contemporary language usage.

While a conceptual definition conveys the researcher's perspective on a given concept, it does not specify the manner in which the variable is to be observed and/or measured and does not describe the steps the researcher must take to gather the required information.

An operational definition assigns meaning to a variable and describes the activities required to measure it. That is, it describes how the variable is to be observed and measured and can thus be manipulated. The operational definition should be so specific that if the study were replicated, another researcher would be able to construct the measurement techniques exactly.

Bless, Higson-Smith and Sithole (2013) suggest three types of operational definitions for a hungry person:

1. A person who has been deprived of food for 24 hours.
2. A person who can eat a loaf of bread in less than ten minutes.
3. A person whose blood sugar is lower than a specified level.

Each definition gives a precise indication of what the researcher needs to do or observe to identify the phenomenon of a hungry person. They can then choose the definition that best fits a particular situation.

Similarly, the operational definition of 'obesity' is a body mass index (BMI) of more than 30 kilograms per square metre. BMI is the mass in kilograms divided by height in square metres. This definition enables anyone investigating the phenomenon to assign the same meaning to the term because it provides specificity.

An operational definition may be influenced by the unavailability of direct information, or the need for information to be obtained through secondary sources. Operational definitions may also be unique to particular research scenarios. For example, if a researcher is unable to obtain demographic data, they can determine it by studying employment level, educational level, income, material possessions and areas of residence.

Research proposal

Sometimes referred to as the 'research protocol', the research proposal is a written statement or plan of the research design which must be submitted to gain approval for the study to proceed. It presents the project plan to demonstrate that the researcher is capable of successfully conducting the proposed research. The researcher can also use it to obtain permission for postgraduate study or to obtain funds needed for the study.

Research ethics committees, managers of institutions, colleagues and supervisors scrutinise the proposal for methodological or ethical problems. Critical appraisal of proposals is also conducted to select the best studies for funding by local, private, governmental, national or international organisations and agencies. The researcher can begin the data-collection process when the proposal is accepted. While the proposal explains how the research will be conducted, it can be adjusted if new insights are acquired (particularly in qualitative research).

The proposal must demonstrate that the study is based on theory, and that it is methodologically sound, practically organised and logical. It should also indicate how it will contribute to the knowledge base in the field of interest. The proposal's compilation also helps the researcher to clarify and refine the research process.

The way in which the proposal is organised varies, but some elements are fairly common. Headings are less important than addressing the 'what', 'why', 'how', 'who', 'where' and 'when' aspects of the study. Every aspect must be clearly articulated and provide the relevant facts in a concise, logical and systematic manner.

The researchers should ask these ten questions when writing a research proposal:
1. What will I research?

2. Why am I undertaking this study?
3. What are the study's aims and objectives?
4. What are the research questions or hypotheses?
5. What are the ethical implications?
6. How will I collect the data?
7. Who will be involved?
8. Where will I conduct the study?
9. When will I conduct the study?
10. How will I interpret the data?

An example of a proposal outline follows. You can adjust it according to the type of study you are conducting or to the specific requirements necessary for obtaining permission to commence or based on the requirements of a potential funder of grants. Although each institution has its own requirements in terms of format, the outline of the proposal should comprise these basic elements:

- The researcher's personal details, including their CV. In the case of a degree study, the study supervisor's information is also required.
- Proposed study title
- Abstract
- Introduction (containing an overview of the broader topic or area of interest to contextualise the study)
- Background (introducing the more detailed discussion of the research problem and questions, including the rationale for the study and some literature review on the topic)
- Aim and objectives (including the problem statement and purpose statement)
- Demarcation of the field of study
- Research methodology, including the design, population and sample, data collection and data analysis
- Significance (thus persuading the reviewer of the value and importance of the study)
- Ethical considerations
- Rigour of the study (trustworthiness, validity and reliability)
- Potential limitations
- Project outline (including the resources that are available and those that are needed to conduct the study, as well as the organisational plan, the work plan, the schedule and the financial plan)
- List of references.

The research proposal forms an integral part of the research process, and a good research proposal serves as a working document for the study. Key principles for critically appraising a proposal include the following steps:

- Read and critically appraise the entire proposal to examine the quality of all aspects of the proposal.

- Examine the lay-out of the proposal in terms of the organisation and presentation of the content (including the editorial aspects).
- Examine the significance of the study for the particular field within which the study will be conducted.
- Examine the explanation of the type of study (approach, design) and the steps that will be followed (methods).
- Identify the strengths and weaknesses of the study. Be objective in doing this and remember your role as reviewer and not supervisor or co-researcher. Some reviewers may think they have to find mistakes and make suggestions for changes, while others may compliment a proposal excessively.
- Provide a rationale for the critical appraisal comments. Give specific examples for improvements or changes. Give specific reasons when complimenting the study.
- Provide guidance and reference where a researcher has missed important literature on the topic. A researcher might not have included leaders in that particular field of study in the proposal's literature review/background to the study.
- Assess the usefulness of the outcomes of the study, for example, where guidelines will be developed for practice.

The review process of a proposal is an important step in ensuring the scientific value of a study.

Summary

In this chapter, we focused on the transformation of a broad, general problem into more manageable, researchable problems. We explored the process of stating the purpose of the study and formulating objectives, questions or hypotheses. Having addressed the identification and definition of different types of variables, we explained the preparation of a research proposal and its significance as the initial step in the broader research process. We also provided some key aspects to consider when appraising proposals.

Exercises

1. Select and read a research article from a research journal then answer the following questions:

    (a) Is the research problem formulated as a question, an objective or a hypothesis?

    (b) Is the purpose of the study clearly stated? If so, what is it?

    (c) Does the research problem have independent and dependent variables? Identify each of them.

    (d) Are the variables operationally defined?

2. Formulate two empirical and two non-empirical research questions.

3. Identify extraneous variables and suggest ways of controlling or limiting them.

4. Identify the independent and dependent variables in the following statements:

    (a) The job turnover rate and job dissatisfaction levels of graduate healthcare professionals who have worked in the field for less than two years are higher than for those who have worked longer than two years.

    (b) There is an inverse relationship between the number of online lectures attended by first-year students and the degree of anxiety during examination.

    (c) Obese teenagers have lower levels of self-esteem than teenagers who are of normal weight.

5. Formulate an operational definition for each of the following variables: nurse, pain, stress and adherence.

6. Select a research topic and draft a research proposal seeking permission to conduct the study.

7. Explain the importance of a research proposal.

8. Should you be the reviewer of the proposal drafted in question 6, what are the key aspects that you will look out for?

Quantitative research

Quantitative research focuses on precise measurement and quantification when investigating a phenomenon. This chapter focuses on the most common quantitative research designs and their underlying principles. The research design stems from the research question or hypothesis, and from the study's purpose. It is the set of logical steps the researcher takes to answer the research question. It forms the 'blueprint' of the study, and determines the methodology used to obtain sources of information (such as participants, elements and units of analysis), to collect and analyse the data, and to interpret the results.

Theoretically, every research question has one specific research design which validates the research findings. However, even the best theoretical design might prove impractical or even impossible in a given circumstance. Researchers choose designs which fit the research purpose, and which are compatible with resources available to them, such as time, funding, sources of information, ethical considerations and personal preferences.

Important concepts and principles in quantitative research designs

The purpose of scientific research is to provide ample evidence regarding the research problem investigated. Several underlying principles are considered when planning and conceptualising a study: understanding their meaning (and those of associated concepts) is critical in selecting a research design.

Rigour

Gray, Grove and Sutherland (2017: 36) describe rigour as 'striving for excellence in research', which in turn implies discipline, attention to detail and meticulous accuracy. It refers to critical aspects of, and is underpinned by, the steps in the research process, and requires scrutiny of each. Researchers make methodological decisions that affect the rigour of a study. Therefore, rigour demands a systematic approach to the research design, and an awareness of the importance of interpretation (rather than relying on assumptions or perceptions). Data are collected systematically, objectively and thoroughly, and are analysed and interpreted in a manner which minimises contamination and enhances accuracy. Detailed and meticulously kept records of collected data are important.

A check on the validity of the study's findings, and the ability of other researchers to yield the same results using the same processes and methods to reach the same conclusions, are further features of rigour (Bowling, 2005; Gray, Grove & Sutherland, 2017). Another is precision: the concise expression of a research problem, and the detailed development of the research design ensure accuracy, detail and order. For example, the use of a cardiac monitor to measure and record the heart rate of a patient admitted to a medical ward, instead of palpating a radial pulse manually and then recording the rate on a data sheet, ensures precision.

Causality

'Causality' refers to the causal relationship between variables, that is, 'some things have causes, and causes lead to an effect' (Burns & Grove, 2020). 'Multicausality' refers to the relationship between variables in which a number of interrelating variables can be involved in causing a particular effect (Gray, Grove & Sutherland, 2017).

An example of causality could include the concentration of fluoride in drinking water and the number of cavities in children's teeth. Pregnancy causing weight gain in women is another example. Causality is also a philosophical issue, which recognises that most phenomena are determined by a variety of conditions. For example, the concentration of fluoride in drinking water causes cavities in children's teeth, but a number of other factors may also cause it. Health researchers usually explore all factors which increase the probability of an effect occurring.

Probability

'Probability' refers to relative (rather than absolute) causality. Quantitative researchers use a probability orientation when designing studies which examine the probability of a given effect occurring under specific circumstances. They recognise that while a particular cause will probably result in a specific effect, it may not produce that effect each time. Terre Blanche, Durrheim and Painter (2016) refer to probability as a concept that involves drawing conclusions about how the world works or what the world looks like. For example, when investigating compliance with treatment, the researcher may examine the effects of multiple variables on compliance. The circumstances affecting compliance may include the education of the patient (about the importance of compliance and the side-effects of the medication), the patient's age and the support extended by family members. Compliance with treatment may vary in relation to a changing set of circumstances.

Bias

'Bias' is an influence which produces an error or distortion that may affect the quality of evidence in both quantitative and qualitative studies. Bias can occur at any step of the research process. When it does, this does not necessarily signal that the researcher caused it (either intentionally or unintentionally), but could be due to problems which occurred as the study evolved and progressed.

Bias can result from a number of factors, and these need to be considered during the study's planning phase. Polit and Beck (2021) cite the following:

- **Participants' lack of openness or impartiality:** in an effort to present themselves in the best possible way, participants sometimes distort their disclosures or behaviour – consciously or subconsciously.
- **Researcher subjectivity:** the researcher's experiences, expectations or hypotheses may skew information – intentionally or unintentionally – in a specific direction. Bias can be induced by communicating their expectations with participants.
- **Sample imbalances:** these can occur when an incorrect sampling approach is adopted, or when there is poor retention of participants. This factor is discussed in more detail in Chapter 10.
- **Errors in data collection:** this occurs when inadequate means are used to capture key concepts. For example, an inaccurate scale used in a study investigating obesity in older persons may exaggerate, or underestimate, the real problem.
- **Inadequate design:** the design does not facilitate an unbiased answer to the research question or does not address the purpose of the study.
- **Incorrect implementation:** the design and methods are flawed owing to careless implementation.

Both the researcher and research consumer are responsible for reducing or eliminating bias. Methodological processes should be scrutinised accordingly and known biases should be considered when interpreting a study's findings. Various strategies can be used to eliminate or minimise bias, thereby strengthening the rigour of a study. Triangulation is one of the most important in minimising bias.

Triangulation

'Triangulation' is the use of multiple sources, or referents, to draw conclusions about what constitutes the truth about a phenomenon, and to clarify and understand the phenomenon (Polit & Beck, 2021). Triangulation is based on the assumption that any inherent bias in a particular data source (whether originating from researcher or method) is neutralised when used in conjunction with others. Although triangulation may increase a study's validity, it should not be used as a substitute for rigour. Triangulation can be achieved through a variety of techniques:

- **Researcher triangulation:** the use of more than one researcher in a single study. The researchers could be from different disciplines, with different levels of expertise. All of them should play prominent roles in the study to achieve intersubjective agreement.
- **Data triangulation:** the use of multiple means of data collection as well as sources such as interviews, observations, questionnaires and diary entries.
- **Theory triangulation:** the use of multiple theories or perspectives to interpret a single data set.
- **Methodological triangulation:** the use of multiple or mixed methods to study a single topic. For example, using both qualitative and quantitative methods in a study.
- **Analysis triangulation:** the use of two or more analytical techniques to analyse one data set.

Basic and applied research

When conceptualising research, the researcher needs to decide whether they want to expand on fundamental knowledge or to solve specific problems. There are thus two categories of research: basic and applied.

Basic research (also called 'academic' or 'pure' research) is research that is aimed at gaining a better understanding of a topic, phenomenon or basic principles of nature. The primary focus is on the advancement of knowledge rather than solving a specific problem. Basic research therefore tends to enhance, or expand on, fundamental knowledge. It is used to support or reject theories by explaining social relationships. For example, a study on the performance of nurses working in primary healthcare clinics in relation to their qualifications would constitute basic research. The findings would have implications for the quality of care and practice, but the study would not attempt to solve a problem. Although this study would be primarily explanatory in nature, it could also be exploratory, descriptive and explanatory. Or, for example, a study on the impact of alcohol consumption on the brain would be regarded as basic research. A study of this nature would not provide a solution to the problem of alcohol consumption and its effect on the brain.

Basic research is also used to interpret changes in communities in order to introduce new scientific knowledge or ideas about societies (Polit & Beck, 2021). One of the advantages of basic research is that it creates a basis for knowledge application and provides insight into social problems, areas of research or policies. The main disadvantage of basic research is that the knowledge acquired sometimes does not offer short-term practical solutions.

Applied research attempts to solve specific problems or, if necessary, to make specific recommendations. It usually focuses more on particular problems and their short-term solutions, rather than on theory. Applied research is generally descriptive in nature, and its main advantage is that it can be applied immediately after the study's findings are obtained (Polit & Beck, 2021). Applied research is therefore problem-orientated and directed at a defined end. Researchers aim to increase what is known about a problem with the aim of creating a better solution. The problem is often needs-based with a particular solution in mind. For example, a study determining the healing aspects of a particular traditional herb for patients who are HIV positive constitutes applied research. The study's implications for practice include emphasising health education to improve safe use of traditional medicine in patients who are HIV positive.

Results obtained through basic research are often reported in technical scientific language, because the data is primarily meant for dissemination among scientists. Results obtained through applied research should be comprehensible to the person requesting the research or to the profession utilising and implementing the research findings. The translation of knowledge gained through scientific research is important. Knowledge translation increases the use of evidence within a variety of contexts related to policy and practice. A variety of knowledge translation toolkits can be found online. The 1 : 3 : 25 format refers to the one-page 'take-home message' (written in simple language), the three-page executive summary, and the 25-page research report. These formats are used to package a study's findings for specific audiences.

Time dimension in research

An essential factor in research is time. It is necessary to determine beforehand how much time is required for obtaining data. The study may take place at a particular time (and would thus be cross-sectional) or may extend over a long period (and would thus be longitudinal). A study can also be classified according to the time at which the data is collected: that is, prospectively or retrospectively.

A **cross-sectional study** is non-current in nature and is done at a specific point in time. All the information on a specific topic is collected at the same time, from the same participants. These studies are limited to a specific time period and focus on a specific phenomenon or problem. The status of the phenomena or a description of the relationships between phenomena at a fixed point in time is investigated – for example, a study on the knowledge, attitudes and perceptions about the effect of the Covid-19 pandemic on the academic performance of university students. Cross-sectional studies are often more manageable and cost-effective than longitudinal ones, as well as less time-consuming. They are thus the most frequently selected by healthcare professionals. The confounding variable of maturation, resulting from the elapsed time, is not present. One of the disadvantages is that they cannot include changes in social processes – and represent only those which occurred during the period when the data were collected. Determining causality is not a purpose of these studies. Cross-sectional studies can be exploratory, descriptive or explanatory in nature, with descriptive studies frequently yielding the best results (LoBiondo-Wood & Haber, 2014).

A **longitudinal study** is conducted over an extended period of time. Data are collected from one sample at different points in time. In this way potential reasons for changes in variables are investigated. Longitudinal studies use continuous or repeated measures to follow particular individuals over extended periods of time – often years or decades. An example of a longitudinal study would be the effect of a keto diet lifestyle on adults. The researcher may measure weight, intake of carbohydrates, emotional effects of the diet and social implications over a period of time.

Polit and Beck (2021) identify the following situations as those which require longitudinal research:

- **Carrying out time-related processes:** when the researcher wants to study phenomena that change over time like physical growth, habitual relapses or occurrences, and learning.
- **Describing time sequences:** the sequences of phenomena could be relevant or important. If a researcher hypothesises that lockdown regulations during a pandemic cause depression, it would be important to determine whether the depression had not preceded the lockdown period or the pandemic.
- **Making comparisons about change over time:** for example, an exploration of the social behaviour of identical twins who were enrolled in boarding school when going to high school.
- **Enhancing research control:** collecting data at multiple points to enhance the interpretability of the results.

Longitudinal studies are predominantly descriptive and explanatory in nature and are used mainly in applied research. One advantage of this type of study is that it can point out specific tendencies with great certainty, thereby enabling researchers to make forecasts. While often more complex and expensive than the cross-sectional study, it is more indicative of social change. Polit and Beck (2021) point out that longitudinal studies sometimes constitute the only way of highlighting specific characteristics of variables, as well as their causal relationships. There are several types of longitudinal designs, including panel studies, follow-up studies, tracer studies and cohort studies.

In **prospective studies**, data about a presumed cause are collected first, with the effect or outcome being measured afterward. These studies can be cross-sectional or longitudinal. Prospective studies usually yield better quality evidence than retrospective ones. An example of a prospective study is the effect of patients' smoking habits on their recovery after contracting the coronavirus. Patients who smoked before falling ill with the coronavirus can be compared with those who never smoked before in terms of dependency on oxygen therapy, discomfort, a need for medical intervention and adverse recovery.

Retrospective studies include those in which data are collected on an outcome occurring in the present and then linked retrospectively to determinants which occurred in the past. The researcher commences with an effect and works backwards to determine the past associations with this effect. These studies are typically cross-sectional. An example of a retrospective study would be a study that investigates the effects of radiation on factory workers, by determining their health status after retirement.

Classification of research designs

While many ways of classifying and describing research designs have been proposed, no single classification is entirely satisfactory. The same terms are often defined differently by different writers, sometimes making it difficult for the researcher to determine that which is most useful.

In quantitative designs a basic distinction is made between experimental and non-experimental designs. In experimental research the researcher actively introduces an intervention or treatment, while in non-experimental research they collect data without introducing treatment or making changes and are, therefore, a bystander (Polit & Beck, 2021). Table 8.1 refers.

Table 8.1 Quantitative designs

Experimental	Non-experimental	Non-traditional
• True experimental designs ○ Pre-test–post-test control group designs ○ Post-test-only control group designs ○ Solomon four-group designs ○ Factorial designs	• Descriptive designs • Survey designs ○ Simple survey ○ Longitudinal survey ○ Developmental survey • Comparative designs • Correlation designs • *Ex post facto* designs • Retrospective designs	• Case studies • Historical studies • Methodological studies • Meta-analysis • Secondary analysis • Evaluation • Needs assessment • Action studies • Philosophical studies

Experimental	Non-experimental	Non-traditional
• Quasi-experimental designs • Time-series designs • Pre-experimental designs • One-shot case study designs • One-group pre-test post-test designs	• Prospective designs • Path analysis designs • Predictive designs	

Source: Based on Bowling (2005); Burns & Grove (2020); Roestenburg et al (2021); LoBiondo-Wood & Haber (2014); and Polit & Beck (2021).

Experimental designs

Experimental designs differ from non-experimental ones primarily because the researcher can control the action of the variables being studied. The researcher manipulates the action of the independent or causal variable(s) and observes and measures the action or outcome on the dependent variable(s). Two sets of variables are thus used. Experimental research seeks to determine a relationship between these two sets of variables.

Experiments are concerned with testing hypotheses and establishing causality, and clinical practice often requires evidence generated from experimental research. However, many factors limit the extent to which purely experimental designs can be used in health sciences research – the most notable being human nature and naturalistic settings. Studying people usually limits the researcher's control over the independent and extraneous variables involved.

True experimental designs

For an experiment to qualify as true, three conditions are necessary:

1. **Manipulation.** This term signifies that the independent variable, which may be an event, an intervention or a treatment the researcher expects to affect the dependent variable, is controlled by the researcher. In other words, the researcher manipulates the independent variable to assess or measure its impact on the dependent variable. It is the effect of this manipulation which is measured to determine the result of the experimental treatment on the dependent variable. For example, the researcher could introduce an intervention, such as an educational programme or a treatment, to some participants and withhold it from others. They then observe the effect of the intervention or lack thereof. The researcher decides what is to be manipulated: for example, the type of educational programme, to whom the manipulation applies, when the manipulation is to occur and how the manipulation is to be implemented.

2. **Control.** This refers to rules imposed by the researcher to decrease the possibility of error, and to increase the probability that the study's findings are an accurate reflection

of reality, and that scientific knowledge is obtained in a controlled manner (Gray et al, 2017). The researcher must be able to exercise control in the experimental situation by eliminating actions of variables apart from the independent ones. They can achieve this by manipulating, randomising, blocking, matching and carefully preparing experimental protocols, or by using control groups.

3. **Randomisation.** A true experimental design requires the researcher to assign participants to experimental or control groups randomly. Random assignment means that each participant has an equal chance of being placed in any of the treatment groups. The primary function of randomisation is to secure comparable, equalised groups with respect to extraneous variables. Compared to other control methods, randomisation has the advantage of controlling all possible sources of extraneous influence, without any conscious decisions on the researcher's part about which variable needs to be controlled. The assumption is that if this is done, the differences in the groups will result from the manipulation of the independent variables, and not from characteristics in the participants that the researcher has not measured (and may not even know about). Randomisation is therefore the most effective method of controlling individual confounding variables (Polit & Beck, 2021).

4. To achieve randomisation, the researcher first identifies an entire, accessible group of participants, then randomly divides this group into two or more subgroups (depending on the chosen design), using random number tables, coin flipping or other techniques (these are explored in Chapter 10).

There is often confusion about the two terms 'randomisation' or 'random assignment' and 'random sampling'. Randomisation (random assignment) is the assignment of study participants to groups in an experimental study. Random sampling, however, refers to a method of selecting people for a study (Polit & Beck, 2017; Burns & Grove, 2020; Gray, Grove & Sutherland, 2017).

Basic true experimental designs are discussed below.

Pre-test–post-test control group design

In this design, participants are randomly assigned to two groups: the experimental group and the control group. Both groups are measured in a pre-test at the beginning of the study. The experimental group is then subjected to the event or intervention, and both groups are measured again. The researcher compares pre-test and post-test scores of the experimental group, as well as the post-test scores of the control group, in order to assess whether the event or intervention made any difference to the experimental group's scores.

For example, a researcher is interested in determining the value of an anti-drug programme for teenagers. The teenagers are given a pre-test on the use of drugs, then exposed to the anti-drug programme, after which they are given a post-test on the use of drugs. They randomly assign teenagers to experimental and control groups, and pre-test both groups on their attitudes towards drug use. The experimental group watches a video, while the control group is given written information similar to that covered in the video. Both groups are post-tested on their knowledge of drug use. The researcher compares the differences between the post-test scores of the two groups. Whatever happens to the experimental group also happens to the control group, except for the 'treatment' tested (video versus written information).

Owing to randomisation, it is expected that the two groups will be equivalent at the pre-test phase. However, it is possible for them to differ, in which case the researcher takes the difference in the pre-test into account when comparing the post-test results. This design allows the researcher to measure the effects of history, maturation and regression on the mean (this is discussed in more detail later in this chapter).

Post-test-only control group design

In this design there is no pre-test. It is useful in situations where it is not possible to obtain a pre-test measure (there are many instances where it may be inappropriate or impossible to pre-test before the independent variable is manipulated). The post-test-only control group design is not an appropriate means of measuring change. For example, a researcher wishes to study the effect of a particular intervention on the incidence of post-partum depression following a caesarean section. It would be inappropriate to develop and induce a postpartum depression pre-test. However, a random sample of caesarean section patients undergoing the same treatment, emotional support and anaesthesia could be randomly assigned to control and experimental groups, and their possible postpartum depression or mental state could be tested.

Solomon four-group design

This design combines the two preceding designs. Participants are randomly selected from a population group, then randomly assigned to four other groups. This design is more complex owing to these four groups, because two groups receive pre-tests and two groups do not. Administering a pre-test may in itself influence the outcome of the experiment (the post-test scores). By combining the pre-test–post-test control group design with the post-test-only control group design to form the Solomon four-group design, the researcher can control the pre-test's effect.

The Solomon four-group design is considered to be a powerful experimental tool because it minimises threats to internal and external validity, and controls the reaction effects of the pre-test. Any differences between the pre-test–post-test groups and the post-test-only groups can thus be more confidently associated with the experimental intervention.

The design is frequently used in health sciences research to study intervention combinations. However, some disadvantages include the fact that it requires a large sample population, and that the data's statistical analysis is complicated.

Randomised control trials

The randomised controlled trial (RCT) is a type of experimental design which intends to evaluate the efficacy of intervention, and to establish a reliable cause–effect relationship. The following elements characterise this design:

- **Selection criteria.** To ensure groups are comparable with regard to all characteristics which may influence the study's outcome, they are selected according to pre-specified inclusion and exclusion criteria.
- **Random sampling.** Where randomisation is done to ensure all participants have an equal chance of being included in either the experimental or control group, random sampling is done before assignment to groups commences.
- **Control.** The researcher introduces control of the experimental situation to eliminate threats to validity by using one or more controls. One control is to use a control group assigned through randomisation.
- **Double-blind procedure.** Neither the researcher nor the participants should know to which groups participants have been assigned.
- **Intervention protocol.** Intervention procedures are standardised to ensure every participant receives the intervention in exactly the same way.
- **Crossover design.** Participants can be re-assigned to the other intervention in a trial, and the responses to different interventions could then be compared.
- **Intention-to-treat analysis.** Participants' responses are analysed within their groups.
- **Effect size.** Intervention and non-intervention outcomes are compared.

Clinical trials may be carried out simultaneously in multiple geographical locations to increase the sample size and resources, and are referred to as 'multi-centred RCTs'. Randomised controlled trials take place in the clinical environment: for example, measuring the effect of a combination of aloe vera gel and mild soap versus mild soap alone in preventing skin reactions in patients undergoing radiation therapy (Olsen, Raub, Bradley et al, 2001).

Factorial designs

Factorial designs allow researchers to simultaneously test effects of more than one independent variable in the same experiment. The independent variables are referred to as 'factors', and both their individual and combined effects can be measured. Typical factorial designs usually incorporate a 2×2 factorial or a 3×3 factorial, but any combination is possible. The first number refers to the independent variables, while the second refers to the levels of intervention. For example, types of therapy – individual counselling ($y1$) or group counselling ($y2$) – can be factors, while lengths of intervention – brief counselling ($x1$), intermediate counselling ($x2$) or long-term counselling ($x3$) – can be levels of intervention. This would yield a 2×3 factorial design and participants would be randomly assigned to one of six combinations, or cells, that would result from this design.

The researcher could therefore determine whether long-term individual counselling is more effective than short-term individual counselling, or whether individual or group counselling is more effective.

Quasi-experimental designs

A quasi-experimental design is used where an intervention is tested without randomisation. These designs therefore lack the 'signature' of a true experiment, which is randomisation. It is sometimes difficult for the researcher to obtain a control group, whether by randomisation or by matching. These difficulties introduce the need for relaxing some requirements of the true experiment. For example, the researcher may omit a control group for comparison, or, if they use a control group, they may omit randomisation in sampling and assignment to experimental and control groups. The researcher thus uses a quasi-experimental design. The control group is often referred to as a 'comparison group' within the context of this design.

Although many quasi-experimental designs are outlined in research literature, two of the most frequently encountered designs are discussed below.

Non-equivalent control group design

This basic design is the most widely used in health sciences research. While similar to the pre-test–post-test control group design, there is no random assignment of participants to experimental and comparison groups. Instead, the researcher selects two similar groups. For example, they choose a group of hypertensive patients attending the cardiology out-patients' clinic at one hospital in Johannesburg and another attending the cardiology out-patients' clinic at another hospital in Johannesburg. The experimental intervention is administered to one group (the experimental group), while the comparison group receives no intervention, or an alternative intervention. The biggest threat to internal validity is selection bias (explained below). Babbie and Mouton (2021) and Grove, Burns and Gray (2013) point out that it is preferable to use a non-equivalent control group than no comparison group at all.

Time-series design

In this design, the researcher collects data on the dependent variable from the experimental group at set intervals, and both before and after the introduction of the independent variable. No control group is used for comparison. The data collected prior to, and after the introduction of, the independent variable are compared for differences in the dependent variable. For example, the researcher assesses the pain levels of a group of patients with lower back pain. After three weeks of pain assessment (01, 02, 03), participants are taught a particular exercise to alleviate their lower back pain. During the next three weeks, pain levels would again be measured (04, 05, 06). The results of this study help the researcher to determine if the pain persists, if the exercise is effective in reducing pain, and, if so, whether the efficacy persists.

This design's advantages lie in the repeated data collection over periods of time before and after the introduction of the independent variable. Participants act as their own control, providing an indication that the independent variable could be responsible for observed change in the dependent variable.

Pre-experimental designs

These designs have many disadvantages, and the researcher has little control over the research. Included among them are one-off case studies and one-group pre-test–post-test designs.

Problems with experimental designs

Although experimental designs are effective in explaining cause–effect relationships between variables, they are subject to the following limitations that make them difficult to apply to real-world problems:

- A number of variables are simply not amenable to experimental manipulation. For example, the researcher cannot manipulate participants' health history, ages or gender.
- Although many variables can be manipulated, ethical considerations prohibit this.
- For example, it would be unethical for a researcher to withhold treatment from a patient or to expose them to dangerous situations.
- Experimental designs may not be feasible because they require additional funds and can be difficult to conduct in settings such as hospitals or clinics. Access to large samples may also not be possible.
- Experiments are complicated by many sources of bias and errors (threats to internal and external validity) which must be dealt with as effectively as possible to ensure that the research is of a high standard. The researcher must always contend with competing explanations for the obtained results.

Threats to internal validity

'Internal validity' refers to the degree to which an experiment's outcomes can be attributed to the manipulated, independent variable(s) rather than to uncontrolled extraneous factors. Other than the independent variable, any factor which influences the dependent variable constitutes a threat to validity.

Polit and Beck (2021) and Gray et al (2017) have identified several threats to a study's internal validity, including the following:

- **History.** This refers to events, other than the experimental intervention (thus, unrelated to the planned study), that occur during a study – between pre-test and post-test – which may affect the results. For example, in a study determining the effects of an exercise programme on weight loss, some of the patients could take up additional exercise, such as tennis, which may influence the outcome. In a study determining the effects of compulsory community service on the quality of patient care by recent healthcare professional graduates, factors such as staffing changes, new policies or changes in patient intake may significantly affect the quality of care. History is controlled by the simultaneous use of at least one comparison group. Additionally, the random assignment of participants to groups helps to control the threat. In the form of extraneous events, history would be as likely to occur in one group as in another. A time-series design may also help to reduce the effect of unanticipated events on, or normal fluctuations in, dependent variables.

- **Maturation.** This refers to changes which occur within participants over time, and which may affect an experiment's results. Changes include physical growth, mastery of new developmental skills, intellectual maturity, healing following an injury or illness, or stress and anxiety. In general, the longer the experimental intervention, the more difficult it is to rule out maturation's effects. The one-group pre-test–post-test design is particularly vulnerable to this threat.

- **Testing.** One of the difficulties of utilising a pre-test–post-test design is the effect of testing and re-testing. Prior exposure to a test or measurement technique can bias a participant's responses. They may remember previous responses and opt to change them, which would alter the outcome of the study. Particular test effects are boredom (when exactly the same test is repeated), practice (participants learn through repetition to respond to tests) and fatigue (particularly when the test is lengthy). To counter these effects the researcher should reduce the number of times participants are tested, vary the tests slightly (to reduce boredom and practice effects), and use shorter tests to reduce fatigue. The Solomon four-group design counters the effect of pre-tests.

- **Instrumentation.** Instruments may present a threat to validity, particularly when those used to record measurements change over time. The changes can occur when people are the instrument, or when a variety of instruments, physical equipment or measuring scales are utilised. Human observers can gain experience and become more proficient in their ratings, or may become tired and make less-exact observations. Equipment can record inaccurate readings and, with repeated use, may need to be recalibrated to maintain accuracy of measurement.

- **Mortality.** Participants may opt out of a study during data-collection procedures or may pass away during the study. There may be more who leave in one group than in others, causing them to differ. It is also possible that participants who choose to leave or are lost due to death are systematically different from those who remain, and this may result in biased findings. For example, if a large number of participants with low pre-test scores leave or are lost due to death, the average scores on the post-test for the experimental group may be deceptively high. The researcher should design the study so that it is convenient for participants to be involved until the end, and should impress upon them the importance of their continued co-operation. Loss to death, however, cannot be foreseen or changed.

- **Selection bias.** Selection is a problem when differences exist in the way participants are recruited and assigned to groups. Unless each group's participants can be shown to be similar before the intervention, the researcher will find it difficult to attribute causality. They should therefore ensure that participants in all intervention groups are as similar as possible. Random selection and assignment, or matching, decreases the potential threat to validity.

- **Demoralisation.** A feeling of deprivation can occur in control groups when participants realise that they are receiving less-desirable interventions. They may withdraw, give up or become angry. These behaviours are reactions to the intervention and are not caused by it. They can also lead to differences which are not attributable to the intervention.

Threats to external validity

'External validity' refers to the degree to which a study's results can be generalised and adapted for other purposes and settings. Two main questions about external validity need to be answered:

1. With what degree of confidence can the findings be transferred from the sample to the entire population?
2. Will the findings hold true at other times and in other places?

The researcher should consider several threats to external validity, including the following:

- **Reactive effects.** These are a group of related effects which result from participants knowing they are being observed and thus behaving in an unnatural manner. An example is test anxiety. The measuring instrument may increase the arousal levels of some participants and influence their scores accordingly. Indeed, some participants could try to please the researcher by providing results they believe are desired. Others may try to compromise the study in order to see how the researcher reacts.
- **Researcher effects.** These threaten the study results when the researcher's characteristics or behaviour influence participants' behaviour. Examples include verbal or non-verbal cues, facial expressions, clothing, age and gender. Researchers may also exert bias in recording observations such that they produce more favourable results. One way to control for this effect is for the researcher to remain 'blind' to group assignments: that is, the researcher should be unaware of which group is the experimental group and which group is the control. If the researcher as well as participants remain unaware of group assignment, double blinding has been employed.

The **Hawthorne effect** may be a threat to both external and internal validity. It occurs when participants respond in a certain way because they know they are being observed. If participants are unaware that they are being observed, there is no reason for them to act unusually and, more importantly, no reason for the researcher to expect them to do so. This is not always possible, however, particularly in instances where obtaining informed consent is necessary.

The most effective way of countering this bias is to use unobtrusive data collection techniques. This may, in practice, mean collecting data from the participants' daily environments and using techniques that do not require a specific set of skills or unusual apparatus. The onus is on the researcher, however, to show that the effect is caused by the intervention and not simply by the participants' participation in the study.

Non-experimental designs

Where researchers do not intervene by controlling the independent variable, a non-experimental study is conducted, and is therefore an observational study. Non-experimental designs are clearly distinguishable from true experimental and quasi-experimental designs because the setting is not controlled and there is no manipulation of the independent variable (and therefore no intervention). The study is carried out in a natural setting and phenomena are observed as they occur. The main purpose of non-experimental research is to describe phenomena and explore and explain relationships between variables. The lack of experimental control makes these designs less able to determine cause and effect than true or quasi-experiments, but they are useful in generating knowledge in a variety of contexts in which it is difficult, unethical or even impossible to employ an experimental approach.

Variables that are difficult to manipulate, or the manipulation of which is unethical, include birth weight, pain, social support, fear, obesity, alcohol intake, drug abuse, grieving, and physical or emotional illness. In these types of design, the researcher is regarded as a bystander. It is as important for them to obtain valid study results in non-experimental research as it is in experimental research. They thus need to consider the extraneous variables which threaten the validity of non-experimental studies.

While many types of non-experimental designs exist, they can be divided into two broad categories.

Descriptive designs

Descriptive designs are used to accurately portray people's characteristics or circumstances, and the frequency with which they occur. These are used in studies where more information is required in a particular field about certain characteristics through the provision of a picture of the phenomenon on certain situations as it occurs naturally. These designs describe the variables in order to answer the research question, but there is no intention of establishing a cause–effect relationship. They may be used to identify problems with current practice, to justify current practice, to make judgements or determine what other professionals in similar situations are doing, or to develop theories (Gray et al, 2017; LoBiondo-Wood & Haber, 2014). Descriptive research encompasses a variety of designs that utilise both quantitative and qualitative methods.

Descriptive designs are based on the following assumptions:
- The variable exists in the study population as a single variable which is amenable to description.
- There is insufficient literature describing the study population or the variable.
- The study may commence without a theoretical framework, but the researcher should provide a rationale for the study based on a thorough literature review, which could be guided by a conceptual framework.
- Existing studies may provide a rationale and theoretical framework for the study at hand in the case of a known concept.
- In a study where criteria for external validity cannot be met owing to unknown population parameters, the findings cannot be generalised.

Descriptive designs are concerned with gathering information from a representative sample of the population. The emphasis in data collection is on structured observation, questionnaires and interviews or survey studies.

Typical descriptive study

Typical descriptive studies are intended merely to describe a phenomenon. The researcher does not manipulate any variables and makes no effort to determine the relationship between them. In these studies the researcher searches for accurate information about the characteristics of a single sample (participants, groups, institutions or situations) or about the frequency of a phenomenon's occurrence. They should identify, and conceptually and operationally define, the variables of interest. These variables can be classified as opinions, attitudes, needs or facts. They are then described to provide a complete picture of the phenomenon.

An example of an opinion or attitude variable is the response to abortion among healthcare professionals at different educational levels. An example of a descriptive study focusing on needs is an examination of the psychological needs of people grieving the loss of a family member to a car accident. An example of variables that constitute facts is the percentage of patients injured during a fall while hospitalised.

Comparative descriptive study

A comparative descriptive study is designed to describe variables, as well as the differences between two or more groups, to see if, and how, they differ. Descriptive and inferential statistics can be used to analyse the differences. For example, if a researcher wants to investigate the level of self-esteem in abused women, they choose a group of women who have experienced abuse and compare them with another group which have not been abused to see the extent to which they differ in self-esteem. Another researcher is interested in studying the effect of the death of a child on physical and psychological well-being. They proceed by taking two groups as they naturally occur: that is, parents who have lost a child and others who have never lost a child and compare them in terms of physical and psychological well-being while providing detailed descriptive information about them.

Descriptive designs with a time dimension

A researcher plans and conducts a study with a longitudinal design when they wish to examine how variables change over time. This design thus relies on a time perspective because the researcher is concerned not only with the existing status and interrelationship of phenomena, but also with changes that result from elapsed time.

Longitudinal studies allow researchers to collect data at several points in time. For instance, a midwife is interested in investigating the development of maternal bonding with the unborn baby in relation to the first time the mother felt the baby move. She selects a group of women pregnant for the first time and collects data on the bonding process from each participant at the 12th, 24th and 36th week of pregnancy. This provides a longitudinal perspective of the bonding process, but the example can be viewed as a short-term longitudinal study. In some instances, longitudinal studies are long term and can continue for years, making them expensive and demanding in ongoing participant and researcher commitments. There are also many threats to validity that must be considered.

Cross-sectional studies are used to examine data at one point in time: that is, the data are collected on only one occasion with different participants, rather than with the same participants at several points in time. For example, the midwife conducting the study on pregnant mothers now selects equivalent groups of women who are pregnant for the first time and who are at each of the respective points of pregnancy – she thus collects data from a group of participants who are 12 weeks pregnant, from another who are 24 weeks pregnant, and from yet another who are 36 weeks pregnant. She then compares the data from each group using statistical measures.

Correlational designs

Correlational research explores the interrelationships among variables of interest, without any researcher intervention. This is also known as *'ex post facto'*, or 'after the fact' design. Its basic purposes are to describe existing relationships between variables and to determine the relationship between independent and dependent variables. Where a correlation exists, a change in one variable corresponds to a change in others.

In correlational studies there is no manipulation of the independent variable because the phenomenon, or dependent variable, has already occurred. Therefore, correlation does not indicate causation. This type of research may confirm the existence of a correlation, but it is generally an insufficient means to indicate that a causal relationship exists.

In descriptive correlational designs, the researcher attempts to determine and describe the relationships which exist between variables. For example, if a researcher wishes to study the relationship between age and fertility they record the fertility of participants from a variety of age groups, as it is impossible to manipulate age. They then determine the relationship between age and fertility through the use of a statistical test known as the 'correlation coefficient'.

When using a **retrospective** design, the researcher starts with an effect and works backwards to determine the associations with this effect in the past. A classic example is the Thalidomide babies: when large numbers of armless and legless babies were reported in the 1960s, researchers looked for factors which could have been the cause, or which could correlate with the effect. They found that all the babies' mothers had taken Thalidomide, a sedative, during pregnancy, and could thus establish a relationship between the drug and specific birth defects.

In a prospective study, the researcher selects a population and follows it over time to determine outcomes. For example, if a researcher wants to study the impact of chronic back pain and functional impairment on patients' quality of life, they will select a group of patients suffering with chronic back pain and determine their pain and functional impairments. They would then follow up on the cases over a period of time to determine participants' quality of life.

The value of correlational designs lies in the fact that many important research problems cannot be studied by experimentation. Moreover, correlational designs are usually inexpensive, can be done quickly, can use large samples from a given population, and can provide meaningful information about how variables function in relation to one another.

Epidemiological research

Epidemiology is concerned with all health and illness in human populations, and with the factors, including health services, which affect them. It is the study of the distribution and determinants of states of health and illness in these populations. **Epidemiological** research involves the gathering of information on disease/health in groups of people, and on agents causing change or preventing disease or recovery in an environment. A well-known example is that of lung cancer: the relationship between lung cancer and smoking was ascertained by epidemiological research on groups of people with lung cancer, who were compared to groups of people without lung cancer. The research demonstrated that more people with lung cancer had smoked cigarettes than those who had not.

The key elements of epidemiological studies are in their simplest form known as the epidemiological triad, which is the traditional model for infectious disease. The triad consists of an external agent, a susceptible host and an environment that brings the host and agent together. The aims of epidemiological studies are to describe the distribution, the pattern, and the natural history of disease in the general population. Epidemiological studies also aim to identify factors that may cause diseases or affect disease processes or patterns, and to evaluate strategies for the control, management and prevention of a disease.

When conducting epidemiological research, the researcher should pose the following questions:

- Why has this person rather than another developed a specific disease?
- How could a specific disease be prevented?
- Why does a specific disease occur in one season rather than in another?
- Why is a disease more prevalent in this country or region than in another?

The following 'simple' set of questions could also guide the researcher:

- Which disease or condition is present in excess? This question is asked to reflect the need for a sound, common definition of a disease so that like is compared with like. It provides a point of reference for what is 'usual' in order to identify 'excess'.

- Who is ill?
- Where do they live?
- When did they become ill?

The three questions determining the who, where and when (that is, person, place and time) form the basis of descriptive epidemiology. This trio captures the essence of the problem and prompts the next question:

- Why did they become ill? This question determines the causes of the epidemic.

The purpose of epidemiology can be summarised as follows:

- description of the health status of populations – who is becoming ill, where and when
- causation – what is causing the problem(s)
- evaluation of interventions – testing possible solutions to try to resolve or reduce the problem
- natural history and prognosis – the course and outcome of the disease, both in individuals and in groups to make public health judgements (Webb, Bain & Pirozzo, 2005).

Epidemiological process

Having evolved from the problem-solving process, the epidemiological process provides a framework for investigating health-related problems, obtaining new knowledge, and planning, implementing and evaluating specific interventions. These processes require critical thinking skills and reasoning abilities. As in any other investigative process, the nature, extent and scope of the problem must be clearly defined.

Epidemiology can be grouped as follows. Quantitative epidemiology deals with numerical descriptions. Descriptive epidemiology uses both qualitative (using words) and quantitative methods. In observational epidemiology the researcher uses observation of human phenomena. Experimental epidemiology is when assessment of the effects of intervention against a disease phenomenon is investigated. The study of mathematical and methodological issues is known as theoretical epidemiology. Epidemiological studies therefore range across three major dimensions: descriptive, analytical and intervention. Epidemiological descriptive studies consist of the description of patterns of disease in populations, and involve the measurement of mortality, morbidity and disability – as always, involving person, place and time. Other typical epidemiological research includes case-control studies, cohort studies, randomised controlled trials, meta-analysis, longitudinal and cross-sectional studies, and correlational studies.

The main uses of epidemiological studies in health sciences comprise:

- investigations of the causes and natural history of disease, with the aim of prevention and health promotion

- measurements of healthcare needs and the evaluation of clinical management, with the aim of improving the efficacy and efficiency of healthcare
- developments in risk screening and diagnostic instruments.

Sources of epidemiological data include 'population-based data' and 'health event data'. Population-based data refer to population statistics such as census, statistics of births and deaths, and morbidity records. These statistics form the basis for accurate descriptions of the population's health status. Health-event data refer to records of vital events in terms of mortality and morbidity.

In short, epidemiological findings play a major role in clinical decision making in terms of assessing, diagnosing and identifying people and populations at risk; planning, implementing and evaluating health services; and developing healthcare policies. For more detailed information of epidemiological research you should consult specific epidemiology sources.

Evaluating quantitative research designs

When evaluating a published research report you may experience difficulty in deciding which aspects of the design make the study useful and important, and which aspects imply flaws which inhibit the use of the findings. Below is a summary of criteria you can use when evaluating research designs.

- Which type of design is used in the study?
- Is the design appropriate in terms of the research question?
- Is the design congruent with the study's purpose?
- What degree of flexibility does the research question require, and how much structure is needed? Was this provided for?
- Is the design suited to the data-collection method?
- Are the research methods clearly described?
- How well does the research design control, or account for, threats to internal and external validity?
- Which threats to validity are not controlled by the research design? How does this affect the usefulness of the results?
- How well does the research design determine causality between dependent and independent variables?

Summary

In this chapter, we presented the basic principles underlying quantitative research, as well as an overview of the most common quantitative designs found in health sciences research, namely experimental designs, quasi-experimental designs, and non-experimental descriptive and correlational designs. We discussed the threats to internal and external validity that a researcher must always take into consideration and attempt to control. We closed the chapter with a summary of the criteria for evaluating a research design, which are directed towards assessing the suitability of the selected design in relation to factors such as the research question and purpose, the methodology and the confounding variables.

Exercises

1. Summarise the most important principles underlying quantitative research.

2. Distinguish between basic and applied research. Provide your own examples of each (you may not draw on those given in this chapter).

3. Give examples of studies (other than those discussed in this chapter) for types of research classified according to time.

4. Differentiate between randomisation and random sampling (consult the chapter on sampling when attempting this question).

5. Answer the following questions based on your knowledge of research design types presented in this chapter:

   (a) Which features characterise each type?

   (b) In what ways do major research designs differ from one another?

   (c) What are the strengths and limitations of each type?

   (d) List specific research questions which could be explored with regard to each design type.

6. Imagine that you want to test this hypothesis: 'Women who have multiple pregnancies are more prone to postpartum depression'. Answer these questions:

   (a) Which research design is most appropriate for this study?

   (b) What are the potential threats to validity in using the chosen research design?

   (c) How could you (as the researcher involved) reduce bias in the study?

7. Differentiate between an experimental and a quasi-experimental design and provide an example suitable for each.

8. Based on your experience as a healthcare professional, identify a problem that would be suitable for an epidemiological study. Explain the steps that would need to be followed.

Qualitative research designs

LEARNING OUTCOMES

On completion of this chapter, you should be able to demonstrate your understanding of:

- the purposes, and some of the distinguishing features, of qualitative research designs
- the aims of qualitative research
- areas in health sciences research where qualitative approaches are particularly useful
- the key elements common to various qualitative research designs
- the nature and function of phenomenology, ethnography, grounded theory and philosophy
- the validity and reliability (trustworthiness) of qualitative research designs
- the relationship of the research design to the research purpose
- doing qualitative research online
- considering mixed methods research
- different types of mixed methods research
- basic principles the researcher must adhere to in mixed methods research

Chapter 8 provided a broad overview of traditional quantitative designs. This chapter covers those of qualitative research designs. Certain questions cannot be answered using quantitative research, and since many problems researchers face can only be studied in real-life scenarios, experimental designs are simply not possible. In these situations researchers ask in-depth questions that require alternative methodologies. Thus, qualitative methodology is used when little is known about a phenomenon, or when the nature, context and boundaries of a phenomenon are poorly understood or defined (Alveson et al, 2021; Burns & Grove, 2020; Creswell & Creswell, 2018; Streubert & Carpenter, 2011).

Various qualitative designs (sometimes referred to as 'qualitative approaches') are used, and there are various schools of thought on specific approaches. This chapter provides an overview of the assumptions on which qualitative research is based, as well as of typical study designs used to answer in-depth questions.

This chapter also provides an overview of mixed methods research. In the previous chapter quantitative designs were discussed and, in this chapter, qualitative designs are discussed. Mixed methods research combines elements of quantitative research and qualitative research to answer a research question. In some studies the research problem cannot be addressed with a quantitative or qualitative design alone and requires the integration of data obtained through both research approaches. For the purpose of this book the authors will only provide an overview of mixed methods research. Specific sources on mixed methods can be consulted for more in-depth information.

Overview of qualitative research

Researchers who wish to explore the meaning, or describe and provide an in-depth understanding of human experiences such as pain, grief, hope or caring, or a phenomenon such as female genital mutilation, would find it difficult to quantify the data. Qualitative methods offer more appropriate and effective alternatives. The research question determines the method, and in this case the research question cannot be 'measured' in quantitative terms. The goal of qualitative research is to understand rather than explain and predict (Alveson et al, 2021; Babbie & Mouton, 2001: 53). The researcher who wants to obtain an insider's perspective needs to stand back and let the research participants' voices be heard. Moreover, the phenomenon often needs to be investigated from various perspectives.

The 'qualitative research approach' refers to a broad range of research designs and methods used to study phenomena. Numerous research designs fall under the umbrella of qualitative research and refer to a collection of methods, each with a specific focus and goal for discovering knowledge. As the name implies, qualitative methods focus on the qualitative aspects of meaning, experience and understanding, and they are used to study human experience from the viewpoint of the research participants in the context in which the action takes place. This is known as an 'emic perspective' or 'insider's view'. The four designs most frequently used in qualitative health sciences research are described below. In these study designs qualitative methods are used to gain access to the study population, to comply with ethical concerns, to collect and analyse data, and to interpret it. A researcher may conduct a descriptive qualitative study that does not necessarily fall into any of the categories mentioned below.

Key features of qualitative research include the following:
- Research is conducted in the real-life situation.
- The focus is more on the process, and less on the product.
- The purpose of qualitative research is an in-depth description and understanding of peoples' beliefs, experiences, perceptions, actions and events in all their complexity.
- The rationale of research is not to generalise the findings, but rather to understand them in context.
- The research is often inductive in nature and generates further questions and hypotheses.

- The researcher is seen as the main instrument, and is subjectively involved in the research process.

Searching the literature in qualitative research

Reviewing the literature is an important step in the research process and is not limited to one specific period in time or way of conducting. Earlier views on the literature review in qualitative research promoted avoiding doing literature review at the beginning of the study completely. However, one cannot enter the new research field without knowing what the field of investigation looks like. Therefore, although with a different approach to exploring the literature, qualitative researchers do engage in some forms of literature review when the study commences. Qualitative researchers approach the literature review differently to quantitative researchers. Qualitative researchers review relevant literature for a preliminary literature review to establish the need for the study, to confirm a lack of evidence about the phenomenon under investigation and to provide guidance for the development of data collection methods. The extensive and in-depth literature review is deferred until after data have been collected and analysed to avoid biasing the analysis and interpretation. The thorough literature review process is sometimes referred to as the literature control, literature integration or exploration of the literature. The literature control places the study's findings in the context of what is already known about the phenomena, and therefore contextualises the findings into the existing scientific body of knowledge. Literature is integrated into the discussion to validate or refute the findings, to gain a better understanding of the findings, and to determine how other researchers have conceptualised and explained similar findings.

Flick (2014) proposes several forms of literature in a qualitative study:

- theoretical literature about the topic of the study
- empirical literature about existing studies in the field or similar to the new study
- methodological literature to support the research design and methods and to guide the processes
- theoretical and empirical literature to contextualise and compare the new study's findings.

These different forms of literature will be reviewed and used in various phases of the study. Style and preferences may vary from researcher to researcher and institutional requirements. It is important that the literature grounds the argument in the study, shows that the findings are in concordance with existing research, and that the findings go beyond or contradict existing knowledge. Exploring the literature requires skilful searches into existing literature. Evidence of a good command of the field under investigation, knowledge of the state of the art of research in the particular field, and an understanding of the problem and methods are required to conduct a review of the literature.

Phenomenology

Phenomenological studies examine human experience through descriptions provided by the people involved, and answer the question: 'What is it like to experience this or that?' These experiences are called 'lived experiences'. The purpose of phenomenological research, then, is to describe what people experience with regard to certain phenomena, as well as how they interpret these experiences. Phenomenologists view the person as integral to the environment. The phenomena make up the world of experiences that are studied as they are and as they occur (Creswell & Creswell, 2018; Leedy & Ormrod, 2010; Polit & Beck, 2021; Streubert & Carpenter, 2011).

In attempting to describe the lived experience the researcher focuses on what is happening in the life of the individual, what is important about the experience, and which alterations are needed – all through the participant's perspective. In this way, the researcher can understand what concepts like 'stress', 'health' or 'caring' mean to the participant. The approach may lead to the development of concepts and themes which can be further developed into interventions to be applied in practice (and often in a participatory manner).

In dealing with people's perceptions or meanings, attitudes and beliefs, and feelings and emotions, phenomenological research places the emphasis on:

- subjectivity rather than objectivity
- description which is more than analysis
- interpretation (understanding) rather than measurement
- agency rather than structure.

The researcher uses several basic actions during the inquiry process:

- **Bracketing.** This involves the researcher identifying and setting aside any preconceived beliefs and opinions they may hold about the phenomenon under investigation. In other words, the researcher identifies what they expect to discover and then deliberately puts the idea aside, thus 'bracketing out' any preconceived ideas so that they can consider every viable perspective. Bracketing is used to mitigate any potential effects of preconceptions that may taint the research process or any activities by the researcher. In phenomenological research it is also called phenomenological reduction, phenomenological epoché or transcendental reduction. This step assists in focusing on the analysis of experience.
- **Intuiting.** This occurs when the researcher tries to understand the lived experience. The process requires them to be open to the meaning that participants attach to the phenomenon and become totally immersed in it (aided by the participants' descriptions). Intuition involves emotional neutrality while maintaining intellectual precision.
- **Analysing.** The researcher repeatedly reviews the data until a common understanding is reached. Analysing entails contrasting and comparing the final data to determine which patterns or themes emerge. If the knowledge is to be relevant and useful to other researchers, it must be understandable and clear, and must detail the relationships that exist.

- **Describing.** The researcher pays careful attention to detail and provides a full description of their findings, together with an 'audit trail' (the particulars of how they collected, captured and analysed the data).

Data-collection techniques include, among others, participant observation in the natural environment, in-depth or unstructured interviews, and diary recording (these are discussed further in Chapter 11).

There are many examples of phenomenological studies in health sciences research. Examples include studies on caring interactions in healthcare professional–patient relationships, existential experiences of illness in a group of immigrant women, story-telling as a teaching strategy, nurse – patient relationships, intercultural communication in healthcare institutions, and a study of living with drug addiction.

Phenomenological research focuses on how life is experienced. The primary concern is not to explain the causes of things, but what is experienced first-hand by those individuals involved. For example, one would not be interested in the extent or reason for homelessness, but rather on how homeless people experience their situation. Phenomenologists focus on:

- seeing things or the world through the eyes of others
- human experiences that are basic, raw and pure, and as directly experienced by others
- the everyday world as the lifeworld of social existence
- social construction of reality as interpreted by others and how they make sense of it
- multiple realities where different people see things differently at different times and in different circumstances
- describing authentic experiences that include the complexity of a situation and the contradictions that populate real life
- suspending common sense beliefs and bracketing their own beliefs temporarily while conducting the research
- exploring matters in depth through mainly unstructured interviews and probing that may become fairly long.

Phenomenological research is suited for small-scale contextual studies. The description of experiences has the potential of unfolding current events, through the feelings and experiences of people about these events. A current example would be the experiences of family relationships during the Covid-19 lockdown period. Through phenomenological research authentic accounts of complex situations could be provided. Using the same example as above, the complexity in family relationships after not being able to visit an elderly parent in a care facility for at least a year could be explored. The humanistic nature of this type of research shows that there is respect for people and their everyday experiences. Because phenomenology does not involve large samples and because of the subjective nature of the research, generalisation is not justifiable.

Ethnography

Ethnography is a qualitative approach which grew out of social anthropology and the study of the culture and customs of groups of people. The focus is thus the social and cultural world of a particular group. Ethnographies are the written reports of a culture from the perspective of insiders (Grove, Burns & Gray, 2013). Ethnography requires spending considerable amounts of time in the setting (or community) in order to observe and gather data of, for example, aspects of the way of life of a particular culture. An underlying assumption is that people's behaviour can only be understood within the cultural context in which it occurs. This differs from phenomenology, which focuses on the meaning of an experience rather than on the role of culture in shaping the experience.

An entire cultural group, or a cultural subgroup, may be studied. The term 'culture' can be used in a broad sense to mean an entire ethnic group, or in a narrower sense, where it is limited to a subunit of a single institution, such as the hospital operating room, the classroom, the doctor's waiting room or a sports team. It could also refer to a culture of a group of people, such a research culture of a particular group.

The researcher is thus able to experience the participants' world – a phenomenon described as 'emic'. Operating from the emic perspective, the researcher examines the language of the culture, learns the organising frameworks and describes the cultural perception of reality from the viewpoint of a member of that culture. In other words, the researcher can obtain, and provide, an insider's view. By contrast, the 'etic' perspective is the researcher's interpretation of the experiences of that culture. As an outsider, the researcher imposes meaning on the cultural experiences of the participants.

Data collection and analysis techniques may vary according to the different forms of ethnography. However, the main techniques employed are participant observation and unstructured interviews. Ethnographers interview people who are most knowledgeable about the culture being studied. These people are commonly referred to as 'key informants'. Other relevant data sources include documents, life histories, films, photographs and artefacts. The researcher writes extensive field notes about them in order to describe the observations they make. Moreover, they use qualitative content analysis to derive patterns and themes from the data, and report the findings in narrative form.

There are many derivatives of ethnography. Leininger developed an interpretation she called 'ethnonursing', which is defined as 'a research method to help nurses systematically document and gain greater understanding and meaning of people's daily life experiences related to human care, health and well-being in different or similar environmental contexts' (Leininger, 1991a: 22). The goal of ethnonursing is to discover nursing knowledge in the ways that it is known, perceived and experienced by nurses and consumers of nursing and health services.

Virtual ethnography, also referred to as 'netnography', is described as being based on the realm of the internet and the virtual world. The techniques of ethnography are transferred to online research where participation is through online communication. Virtual ethnography adapts the traditional ethnography to the study of online cultures and communities formed through computer-based communications (Flick, 2014).

Grounded theory

Grounded theory research is an inductive research approach. Its findings are grounded in the concrete world experienced by the participants and interpreted at a more abstract theoretical level (Grove, Burns & Gray, 2013; Polit & Beck, 2022). Charmaz (2014) explains that grounded theory has a subjective approach to knowledge development due to the involvement in the subjective world of participants. Both researcher and participants contribute to the interpretation of meanings and actions. Charmaz also states that the complexities of particular worlds, views and actions are explored, and that this supplies the how, and sometimes the why, of particular situations. As grounded theory is a qualitative methodology and inductive in nature, the researcher does not begin the research with a preconceived idea. Sheppard (2004) explains grounded theory as an understanding approach which requires the researcher to have an empathetic understanding of the participants' views and context. Polit and Beck (2022) refer to the Glaser and Strauss precepts which state that grounded theory does not begin with a focused research problem. The problem and process rather emerge from the data and are discovered during the study. Other researchers, like Glaser (Polit & Beck, 2022), describe grounded theory as generating concepts and theories that explain and account for differences in behaviour in the substantive area of research rather than describing a detailed and full set of behaviours in substantive contexts. In its simplest form, this theory emerges from data grounded in the observation and interpretation of phenomena. The approach therefore identifies concepts and the relationship between them in an inductive manner. Its purpose is to build theory that illuminates the area of study.

As in the case of ethnography, the process begins in the social and cultural environment. Unlike ethnography, however, grounded theory does not seek to understand culture and cultural processes – reality is instead perceived as a social construct. In grounded theory researchers immerse themselves in the social environment.

Data collection techniques are the same as in most other forms of qualitative research: participant observation and unstructured interviews. Observations are made about the structure and patterns noted in the social environment, and people's interactions are studied through interviews. Document analyses of organisational charts and policies, patient records and other data sources provide additional perspectives in clarifying the social phenomenon.

One of the fundamental features of this approach is that data collection and analysis occur simultaneously. A procedure called 'constant comparison' is used, in which newly collected data are constantly compared to existing data so that commonalities and variations can be determined. An incident is compared with another, one category with another category and one construct with another construct across all observations. Significant incidents or observations are marked or highlighted in the text and assigned codes. These codes are constantly reviewed as new interpretations emerge. The researcher keeps an open mind and uses an intuitive process of interpretation (a process described in greater detail in Chapter 12).

Once the researcher has identified concepts and specified their relationships, they consult the literature to determine if similar associations exist. Despite the diversity of gathered data, the grounded theory approach presumes that it is possible to discover fundamental patterns in all social life. These patterns are called 'basic social processes' (BSPs). Data collection continues until the BSP emerges. The constant comparative process is extremely rigorous in that the researcher has to reflect on categories and must test emerging concepts and relationships many times before being able to make firm theoretical propositions.

Qualitative research using the grounded theory approach has become increasingly popular in the health sciences and is evidenced by the growing number of journal articles and papers presented at conferences. Examples of grounded theory include the studies on trust in the teaching and learning environment, older women's experience of urinary incontinence, the hidden curriculum in a military nursing education context, uninsured African-American men diagnosed with prostate cancer, and the study on the bereavement experience of caregivers.

Philosophical inquiry

Grove, Gray and Burns (2018) explain philosophies as rational intellectual explorations of truths or principles of conduct, knowledge or being that describe different viewpoints on what reality entails, which ethical values and principles should guide our practice, and how knowledge is developed.

The purpose of philosophical inquiry is to perform research using intellectual analysis to clarify meaning, to make values manifest, to identify ethics and to study the nature of knowledge (Burns & Grove, 2019). Research which focuses on philosophical questions is difficult to design and pursue. Many health sciences research textbooks do not include this type of design, yet philosophical questions abound for healthcare professionals.

For example:
- What is nursing/physiotherapy/occupational therapy?
- What are the boundaries of these sciences, and which phenomena belong to them?
- Which thoughts, ideas and values are important to these sciences?
- What is the meaning and purpose of human life, if any?
- How is free will to be interpreted?

- What is the significance of dignity, and what does it mean to be compassionate and caring?

Healthcare professionals confront many philosophical questions relating to ethics, such as obligations, rights, duties, concepts of right and wrong, conscience, justice, intention and responsibility. These questions can be divided into three categories: foundational studies, philosophical analysis and ethical analysis.

The philosophical researcher considers an idea or issue from every possible perspective through exploring the literature, examining conceptual meaning, raising questions, proposing answers and suggesting the implications of those answers. The research is guided by the questions. As with other qualitative approaches, data collection and analysis occur simultaneously. The data sources for most philosophical studies are written materials and verbally expressed ideas. The researcher often explores and debates these ideas, as well as pertinent questions, answers and consequences with colleagues during the analysis phase.

Philosophers primarily engage in **argumentation**. Regardless of whether they formulate analyses of concepts, draw distinctions, discuss assumptions or construct interpretations, philosophers use arguments. Argumentation by analysis, argumentation by interpretation and argumentation by logical structure are philosophers' specialised intellectual tools.

Classical examples of philosophical inquiry are Carper's (1978) study of the ways of knowing in the health sciences; Smith's (1981) idea of health; and Kayser-Jones, Davis, Wiener and Higgin's (1990) ethical analysis of an elder's treatment. More recent studies include the study on selfhood in the context of gender and studies on digital identities and virtual life.

Rigour in qualitative research

Integrity in qualitative research is critical. Reliability and validity of research findings are of great importance in all studies, but in qualitative research they are sometimes viewed with scepticism. Some studies are criticised for lack of rigour, but the criteria used to determine the rigour of qualitative studies tend to be similar to those developed for quantitative studies. This is a mistake, as the processes and outcomes of qualitative research are different from those of quantitative research (Burns & Grove, 2019; Gray, Grove & Sutherland, 2017). Indeed, methods for establishing reliability and validity in qualitative research are not the same as those used in quantitative research: qualitative researchers tend to reject the terms 'reliability' and 'validity' in favour of 'consistency', 'dependability', 'conformability', 'auditability', 'recurrent patterning', 'credibility', 'trustworthiness' and 'transferability' (Corbin & Strauss, 2008; Gray, Grove & Sutherland, 2017; Leininger, 1991; Lincoln & Guba, 1985; Miles, Huberman & Saldana, 2013). This textbook refers to the term 'trustworthiness'.

'Rigour' in qualitative research signals openness, relevance, epistemological and methodological congruence, thoroughness in data collection and the data-analysis process, and the researcher's self-understanding. Polit and Beck (2021) emphasise that the researcher's self-understanding in qualitative research is an interactive process involving the researcher's personal history, values, gender, social class, race and ethnicity as well as those of the participants. The researcher needs to be willing to dismiss preconceived ideas and judgements about the phenomenon and participants, and participate in the research with openness.

Reliability is concerned with the consistency, stability and repeatability of the informants' accounts, as well as the researcher's ability to collect and record information accurately (Creswell, 2013). The underlying issue here, according to Miles, Huberman and Saldana (2013), is 'whether the process of the study is consistent, [and] reasonably stable over time and across researchers'. Qualitative researchers often work alone and need to document their data accurately and comprehensively (leaving a detailed audit trail to check and re-check the consistency in coding the data), to meet regularly with co-investigators and coders for consensus discussions, and to cross-check the analytical framework with emerging codes (Creswell, 2013; Polit & Beck, 2022).

Validity is concerned with the accuracy and truthfulness of scientific findings (Polit & Beck, 2021). Establishing validity requires, first, the determination of the extent to which conclusions effectively represent empirical reality and, secondly, an assessment of whether constructs devised by researchers represent or measure the categories of human experience that occur. In qualitative research, credibility and authenticity relate to internal validity. The researcher asks: 'Are the findings credible to the people I am studying, as well as to my readers?' and 'Do I have an authentic portrait of what I am looking for?'

The two theorists Lincoln and Guba (1985, 1994) propose five criteria for trustworthiness: credibility, dependability, confirmability, transferability and authenticity.

Credibility refers to the truth value of data and interpretations thereof. The following two aspects are important: the study must be conducted in a way that enhances the believability of the findings and the correct methods must be used when conducting the research.

Techniques used to achieve credibility include:
- remaining in the field over a long period of time (prolonged engagement and persistent observation);
- using a variety of sources in data gathering (triangulation);
- peer debriefing (where researchers expose themselves to disinterested peers who probe their biases, explore meanings and clarify the bases for particular interpretations);

- searching and accounting for disconfirming evidence (negative case analysis);
- having research participants review, validate and verify the researcher's interpretations and conclusions (member-checking), which is done to ensure that the facts have not been misconstrued.

Dependability is a further criterion to establish the trustworthiness of the study listed by Lincoln and Guba (1985). It refers to the stability of the data over time and condition, thus to the reliability of the findings. This requires an audit. The inquiry auditor (generally a peer) follows the process and procedures used by the researcher and determines whether they are acceptable (that is, dependable). If dependability is not attained, credibility cannot be claimed.

In order to check dependability, the following aspects must be considered and checked (audited):

- the raw data and how it was collected and recorded
- how data was reduced and synthesised, theoretical notes and transcripts
- reconstruction of the data and the results of the synthesis, structure of the themes, definitions and relationships, integration with the literature
- methodological notes
- filed notes and reflective notes
- information of the data collection instrument and pre-testing.

Questions that could be asked include:

- Are findings grounded in the data?
- Are inferences logical?
- Is the theme/category structure appropriate?
- Can the methodological process be justified?
- What is the degree of researcher bias?
- Would the findings be repeated should the study be replicated with similar participants or the same sample?

Confirmability guarantees that the findings, conclusions and recommendations are supported by the data and that there is internal agreement between the researcher's interpretation and the actual evidence. The objectivity of the findings lies within the potential for congruence between two or more independent researchers (coders) about the accuracy of the data, the meaning and the relevance. This is also accomplished by the incorporation of an audit procedure.

Questions that could be asked include:

- Does the data represent the information provided by participants?
- Has the researcher interpreted the data as it is or through imagination?
- Do the findings reflect the participants' voices?
- Do the findings reflect the conditions of the inquiry and not the biases of the researcher?

Transferability refers to the applicability of the findings to other contexts. For transferability to be possible the researcher must provide sufficient descriptive data that will enable other researchers or other readers to evaluate the relevance of the data for other contexts. For this to be possible a dense (thick) description of the data is necessary to enable others to make a transfer and draw conclusions about whether transfer can be considered as a possibility. The researcher helps to provide a detailed database and description so that someone else can determine whether the study's findings are applicable in another context or setting. In qualitative research transferability and/or 'fittingness' is similar to external validity, which is defined by quantitative researchers as the degree to which the results of a study can be generalised to other settings or samples.

The researcher asks:
- Are the conclusions of the study transferable to other contexts?
- Do they 'fit'?

Authenticity can be established by context-rich and meaningful ('thick') descriptions (Denzin, 1989). The data must convey the feeling tone of the participants' lived experiences. Authenticity is present when readers of the data experience a heightened sensitivity to the issues being depicted. There will be some sense of the emotions, language, experience, mood and contexts of the lives of the participants (Polit & Beck, 2022).

Miles, Huberman and Saldana (2013) provide a detailed description of tactics and strategies that ensure the trustworthiness of a study:
- Check for **representativeness**: The researcher needs to determine whether the behaviour of the people they observe, for example, is present when they are not observing.
- Check for **researcher effects**: The presence of the researcher can affect behaviour.
- To limit this reaction, the researcher should remain on the study site long enough to become familiar with research participants, use unobtrusive methods in dealing with them and seek their input.
- Utilise **triangulation**: Various methods can be used to collect data from sources to ensure confirmability of the findings.
- Weigh the **evidence**: In working with large amounts of data, the researcher looks for evidence that refutes it, as well as that which confirms their conclusions.

Choice of research design

Whether it is traditional or non-traditional, quantitative or qualitative, no particular research design is considered to be more valuable than another. The best design is always one that is most appropriate to the research problem, research question and purpose.

Table 9.1 presents an example of how the choice of design varies in relation to the purpose of the study. The example not only indicates how the choice of research design varies with the purpose, but also demonstrates how at least five research projects can evolve from one problem area (in this case, obesity in teenagers) and how both quantitative and qualitative designs are appropriate, depending, of course, on the study's purpose.

Table 9.1 The problem of obesity in teenagers from community X: research design and purpose

Design	Purpose of study
Descriptive (eg case study or survey)	To describe the dietary patterns of obese teenagers in community X
Correlational	To determine the relationship between compliance with a weight-reduction protocol and successful weight loss in obese teenagers residing in community X
Experimental	To compare the effectiveness of two weight-reduction protocols on the incidence of weight loss in obese teenagers resident in community X
Methodological	To develop and test the reliability and validity of an instrument to measure the influence of dietary patterns on obese teenagers
Exploratory (qualitative eg ethnographic or phenomenological)	To explore how the obese teenagers residing in community X experience their obesity

An introduction to mixed methods research

Mixed methods research refers to a research strategy that combines alternative research approaches within a single study. A deliberate combination of approaches is used with different underlying assumptions and paradigms. The aim of mixed methods researchers is to draw on the strengths of both qualitative and quantitative approaches and to limit the weaknesses in using one single approach. A key feature of mixed methods research is the strength of the methodological pluralism that could lead to superior research (Mitchell, 2018).

Mixed methods research should not be confused with research using multiple methods. An example of multiple methods research would be where multiple quantitative designs are used to answer a research question.

Diverse definitions of mixed methods research exist. Some state that mixed methods research involves the collection and integration of qualitative and quantitative data in a single or a series of studies where mixing can occur at the level of methods (Creswell, 2013), methodology (Tashakkori & Teddlie, 2010), or across disciplines. Tashakkori and Teddlie (2010) refer to the term *mixed model research* when integrating beyond the level of methods. Mixed methods research is therefore an approach where the researcher uses both qualitative and quantitative data in a single study, integrates the sets of data and then draws interpretations based on the strength of both the approaches to answer the research question (Creswell, 2013). Through the systematic integration of both qualitative and quantitative data a deeper understanding of a phenomenon is claimed. The distinct claim in mixed methods research is the *integration* of findings from the qualitative and the quantitative phases.

Mixed methods research can also take on the form of a literature review and is particularly used to generate evidence for complex health and social interventions. Leeman, Voils and Sandelowski (2016: 167) describe mixed methods literature reviews as being 'distinct in that they summarise and integrate findings from qualitative, quantitative, and mixed methods studies via qualitative and/or quantitative methods'.

The philosophical underpinning of mixed methods research is pragmatism (combining positivism and interpretivism). Pragmatism supports the use of different research approaches and methods, and enables a continuous cycle of inductive and deductive reasoning, and where appropriate, abductive reasoning. Abductive reasoning addresses the weaknesses of inductive and deductive reasoning by taking incomplete (sometimes referred to as 'messy') observations from experience and reality to the best predictions of the truth and in some instances, to new theory. Abductive reasoning is similar to deductive and inductive reasoning in that it is applied to draw logical inferences and construct theories. Where a researcher has identified a research problem that cannot be addressed using one approach alone (either by measuring or understanding the phenomenon), both numerical and cognitive reasoning may be combined. The researcher generalises from the interactions between the specific and the general. Abduction focuses on theory generation or modification by integrating existing theory where suitable, to build new theory or adapt existing theory.

Major types of mixed methods designs

The four major types of mixed methods designs are (1) triangulation design, (2) embedded design, (3) explanatory design, and (4) exploratory design. There are several typologies for classifying the four major types of mixed methods designs. **Triangulation design** is the most common design where the researcher aims to gather different though complementary data on the same topic to best address the research problem. In this design the researcher aims at directly comparing and contrasting qualitative findings with quantitative statistical results, validating or expanding results with qualitative data. The **embedded design** is used where one data set provides a supportive, secondary role with an emphasis on the other data set. This design is used where a researcher aims at including qualitative or quantitative data to answer a research question within a large quantitative or qualitative study. The researcher therefore embeds a component of the one research into the other approach. The **explanatory design** is a two-phased design with initial quantitative data where qualitative data is used to build upon the initial quantitative results. Qualitative data is typically used to explain the significance or non-significance of the quantitative results. In this design the researcher starts with the collection and analysis of quantitative data, followed by qualitative data. The **exploratory design**, also a two-phased design, is a design where the findings of the first approach (qualitative) assist in developing the second phase (quantitative). This design focuses on the need for exploration for the following reasons: instruments or measuring tools are not available, variables are unknown or a guiding framework or theory is absent. This design starts qualitatively and is therefore suitable to explore a phenomenon.

The three basic mixed methods designs as described by Creswell and Creswell (2018) are: convergent parallel mixed methods design, explanatory sequential mixed methods design and exploratory sequential mixed methods design. Creswell and Creswell (2018) further refer to an instrument building model of mixed methods design.

Convergent Parallel Mixed Methods

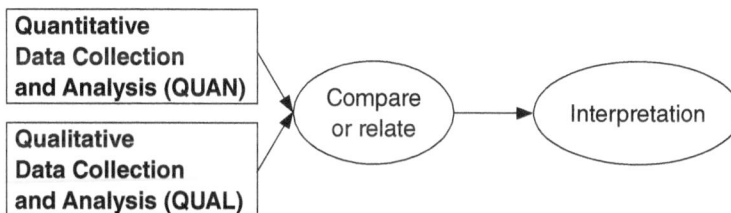

Explanatory Sequential Mixed Methods

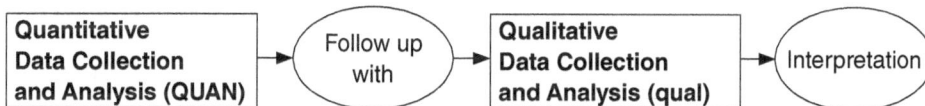

Exploratory Sequential Mixed Methods

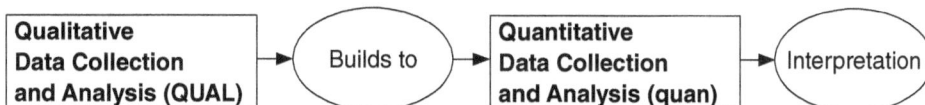

Figure 9.1 Research design: Qualitative, quantitative and mixed methods design

Selecting the type of design will require initially asking certain questions:

- What is the problem I want to investigate?
- What are my research abilities and experience?
- What specific research skills do I have (eg knowledge on statistics or narrative analysis)?
- What resources do I have in terms of time, funding, access to the setting?

Once these questions have been addressed, the decision will further be informed by the following questions:

- What will the timing of the quantitative and qualitative methods be? The timing or sequence refers to order in which the researcher will collect, analyse and interpret the data. The researcher has a choice of two timings for sequential timing: quantitative first, followed by qualitative, or qualitative first, followed by quantitative.
- What will the weighting of the quantitative and qualitative methods be? Weighting refers to the relative priority or importance of the quantitative and qualitative methods. The researcher decides where both the approaches have equal priority or whether one will have a greater priority than the other.
- How will the quantitative and qualitative methods be mixed? Mixing can take place by either integration (merging) of the data or embedding the one set of data into the other.

Implementing the designs will be as follows:

- In the triangulation design (QUAN + QUAL) the timing will be concurrent with usually an equal weighting and data integration.
- In the embedded design (QUAN(qual) or (QUAL(quan)) timing can be concurrent or sequential, with unequal weighting and embedded mixing.
- In the explanatory design (QUAN ⇨ qual) the timing is sequential where quantitative data is collected first, followed by qualitative data collection. The weighting is usually on quantitative methods and the data is then integrated.
- In the exploratory design (QUAL ⇨ quan) the timing is sequential where qualitative data is collected first, followed by quantitative data collection. The weighting is usually on qualitative methods and the data is then integrated.

When a researcher decides to conduct mixed methods research, careful consideration must go into the planning. The questions above could be used to make this choice. Considering the factors that inform your choice must therefore be based on the research problem and how best to address the research question.

It is beyond the scope of this textbook to expand more on mixed methods research. Excellent sources exist that provide detailed information on mixed methods research.

Summary

In this chapter we presented an overview and the distinguishing characteristics of the most common qualitative designs such as phenomenology, ethnography, grounded theory and philosophical inquiry. The trustworthiness of qualitative research was discussed, and an example was given of the manner in which the choice of a research design depends on the purpose. An introduction to mixed methods research was provided, which was meant to open up the thought processes around using both research approaches.

The intention of this chapter was simply to be an introduction. If you wish to do an in-depth study of the designs that we have discussed, you need to explore the texts to which we refer.

Exercises

1. Reflect on your clinical practice and identify a research problem or question for which a qualitative research method may provide an answer. Using the characteristics of qualitative methods, describe how you could present the study.

2. Select one of the two excerpts below and complete the activities which follow.
    Excerpt A: A healthcare professional works in a critical care unit, where many of the patients are terminally ill after contracting the coronavirus. He structures an investigation to determine the grief experienced by family members who are not able to visit their dying family members.

    Excerpt B: A health sciences educator wants to investigate the research culture and practices of postgraduate nursing students.
    (a) Identify the type of qualitative research approach that would be most appropriate for use in the scenario you have selected.
    (b) Identify the sources of data.
    (c) Discuss the researcher's role in the study.
    (d) Briefly identify how data could be recorded and analysed.
    (e) Describe what could be used to add credibility to the study.

3. Propose a topic that could be investigated using virtual ethnography.

4. Select an article from a recent health sciences journal in which a qualitative method was used. Identify the strategies the researcher used to ensure trustworthness.

5. Debate the differences between phenomenology and grounded theory, and explain your choice of design when exploring the lived experiences of elderly adults living in care facilities.

6. Select a topic that you think will be best addressed by mixed methods research. Answer the questions related to deciding on whether mixed methods research will be suitable.

7. Using the same example as in question 6, choose the design and type of mixed methods that will be most suitable.

8. Search for two articles that report on a mixed methods study. Identify the type of design and its suitability to the topic.

Sampling

Having selected and defined the research problem and decided which approach to use to investigate it, the researcher must choose the elements, objects, persons and events from which data needs to be drawn. They therefore need to define the population and sample. The researcher may occasionally study an entire population, but this is likely to occur only when there are a few persons with the characteristics in which the researcher is interested. As a rule, though, the entire population is too large, unwieldy and widespread to be studied directly. The study of each element in the population would take too long and be impractical and costly. The researcher thus works with samples because they tend to provide a more accurate picture of the phenomenon under investigation.

Basic sampling concepts

Research aims to optimise the use of resources in the investigation, and sampling is one way of doing exactly that. 'Sampling' refers to the process of selecting the sample from, or a portion of, a population to obtain information regarding a phenomenon in a way that represents the study population.

Population

A population is the entire group of persons or objects that is of interest to the researcher, and that meets the criteria they are interested in studying (Burns & Grove, 2020; Polit & Beck, 2022). Gray, Grove and Sutherland (2017) describe the term as setting boundaries about the elements or participants. The entire set of elements about which the researcher would like to make generalisations is also called the 'target population' (LoBiondo-Wood & Haber, 2014). For example, if a researcher studies South African patients who have had cardiac surgery, the population is defined as all South African citizens who have had surgery classified as cardiac surgery in a hospital in South Africa. Other examples of populations are all South African men who have undergone traditional circumcision, and all premature babies born in Namibia.

Researchers do not always have access to the entire population, however, and the population they do have access to (and actually study) usually differs in one or more aspects. This population is known as either the 'accessible population' (Grove, Gray & Burns, 2015; Polit & Beck, 2021), or the 'study population' (Padgett, 2017; Struwig & Stead, 2001). While it is improbable that a Western Cape-based researcher in South Africa would be able to find every South African child with congenital heart disease, it may be possible for them to locate those treated at South African tertiary hospitals in the last two years.

The accessible population may not always be available to the researcher if, for example, entry permission is refused by an authority. In this case the researcher must limit the accessible population by adding a characteristic to the defined population, such as restricting the study's setting to tertiary hospitals in the Western Cape. The researcher then plans to generalise their findings to this particular population rather than the entire population. The sample of children treated at tertiary hospitals may be quite different from samples treated at private hospitals, where patients belong to a medical aid scheme. The former group is likely to have a socio-economic background that is different to that of the latter. As a result, conclusions drawn from this sample would probably be invalid as regards the population in private hospitals and are therefore not generalisable to the total population.

It is critical that researchers carefully define and describe the population, and stipulate inclusion criteria. These criteria are also referred to as 'eligibility criteria' or 'distinguishing descriptors' (Polit & Beck, 2021). Researchers should use them as the basis for decisions on whether an individual, element or object would or would not be classified as a member of the population in question. Furthermore, some criteria would lead a researcher to exclude certain elements – individuals, elements or objects – from the population. These criteria are called 'exclusion criteria' or 'delimitations'.

By definition, a sample is a part, or fraction, of a whole, or a subset of a larger set, selected by the researcher. It consists of a selected group of the elements or units of analysis from a defined population. In sampling terminology the element is the most basic unit about which information is collected. In health sciences research the element is typically an individual, but other entities can also form the basis of a sample or population. Examples include: documents, artefacts, blood group, events, groups of people, organisations, behaviours, or any other single measurement unit of a study (LoBiondo-Wood & Haber, 2014). When a researcher includes the entire population in a study, reference is made to a census or all-inclusive sampling.

Sampling frame

The sampling frame is a comprehensive list of the sampling elements in a target population. The sample for a study is drawn from it. Lists of populations, such as membership of a professional nursing organisation, hospital or clinic admission registers, human resource lists, are sometimes readily available. The researcher often prepares a sampling frame by listing all members of the accessible population. This can be a time-consuming task, and the researcher must take care to delineate the population accurately. Inadequate sampling frames which disregard a part of the target population have been the cause of many poor-quality research findings and results. An adequate sampling frame should therefore include all elements of the population under study.

Parameter and statistics

A specific measure or numerical value which relates to the population, such as age, gender, educational level, income or marital status, is known as a 'population parameter'. A **parameter** is a specified characteristic present in each of a population's elements. It is the description summary of a given variable in a population. An example of a parameter is the mean age of pregnant women attending an antenatal clinic. A parameter is thus a measure or value collected from a population which describes the particular characteristic of that entire population.

The corresponding measures, or numerical values or quantities, of a sample (such as 25 years of age, or 60 kg in weight) are referred to as 'sample statistics'.

One of the aims of research is to describe certain characteristics of a target population. Therefore, one of the objectives of sampling is to draw inferences about the unknown population parameters from the known sample statistics by obtaining data.

A representative sample

'Representativeness' means that the sample population should be as similar to the entire population in as many ways as possible. The sample should thus replicate the population variables in approximately the same proportion as they occur. The demographic information the researcher commonly examines includes relationship status, educational level, gender, ethnicity, age and income level, as these tend to influence the study variables. For example, if age and educational level are variables (or population parameters) relevant to the study, then a representative sample will have similar proportions, or representativeness, of the same age groups and levels of education as the target population.

Representativeness is extremely important when the researcher wants to generalise from the sample to the target population by drawing conclusions about the population from which the sample derived.

Sampling error

Sampling error is the difference between a sample statistic and a population parameter. A large sampling error indicates that the sample has failed to provide an accurate representation of the population. Sampling error is not under the researcher's control and is caused by chance variations. It is difficult for the researcher to provide statistics equal to the population parameters they are to estimate, and sampling error is more likely to occur if the population or sample size is relatively small. The larger the sample size, and the more homogeneous the population, the lesser the chance of a sampling error occurring. When the researcher uses careful probability sampling, they can estimate the degree of error statistically.

Sampling error may occur because of the following factors:

- **The chance factor:** One element and not another has been included by chance. These errors can be calculated statistically but can never be completely eliminated. This type of error is not a kind of bias, but rather variability or random variation and occurs by chance.
- **Bias in selection:** Results primarily from the incorrect technique being employed. This kind of bias is often avoidable and may or may not be deliberate. A researcher may, for example, fail to consider the marital status of the participants or they may give incorrect information in this regard. Some segments can be over- or under-represented in a sample. For example, a sample that contains 50 per cent black and 50 per cent white respondents would under-represent the black population and over-represent the white population of South Africa. Bias in selection is therefore a deviation that is not due to chance.
- **Non-response error:** This occurs when, for unknown reasons, an element does not respond to the measurement instrument. Reasons for non-response errors may include issues such as language or reading disabilities, illness and withdrawal from the study, or refusal to provide information. Since these elements are subsequently excluded from the sample, its constitution (and thus representativeness) changes.

Sampling bias

Sampling bias refers to the over- or under-representation of a segment of the population which impacts on the purpose of the study and its validity. It is caused by the researcher and occurs when samples are not selected carefully. Sources of sampling bias can be the time of day or year when the data were collected, the place in which they were gathered, the language used, the extent to which personal views influenced the data, the use of an incomplete or incorrect sampling frame, or the researcher being guided by preference when selecting research participants. In the medical field reference is made to ascertainment bias. Sampling bias limits generalisability of findings as it is a threat to external validity. An example would be where a researcher wants to investigate drug use among school-going teenagers. If teenagers attending high schools are included in the study, the sample will be biased because home-schooling teenagers are excluded.

Sampling approaches

There are two basic sampling approaches: probability (or random sampling), and non-probability sampling.

Probability or random sampling

In the case of probability sampling, the sample is more likely to be representative of the population and to reflect its variations. It implies that all elements in the population have an equal chance of being included in the sample. For example, if professional nurses belonging to a union are the population, then the membership list of the union will be the sampling frame from which the sample will be drawn. Each of the members will therefore have an equal chance of being included in the sample.

Probability sampling also permits the researcher to estimate the sampling error, reduces bias in the sample or sampling, and facilitates the correct use of inferential statistics by the researcher. When the researcher's primary concern in selecting a sample is to obtain findings which can be generalised, a probability sample would be the best choice.

To obtain a probability sample, the researcher must identify every element in the selected population. There must be an available listing of all members of the population, and the sample must be selected from the list at random. The list is the single most important criterion in determining whether probability sampling is possible for a given study. If it is, then one of the common techniques employed in probability sampling may be used, which include: simple random sampling, systematic random sampling, stratified random sampling and cluster sampling.

Techniques or types of probability or random sampling

The selection of an element or unit from a population is referred to as 'random' when each of them has the same chance, likelihood or probability of being chosen for the sample. The probability samples discussed below all use the process of random selection.

Simple random sampling

Simple random sampling is the most basic random sampling technique. Simple random samples are drawn using the basic probability sampling technique. Participants or elements are drawn in a random way from the sampling frame. Each of the elements is listed separately and therefore has an equal chance of being included in the sample.

The main features of a simple random sample are:

- It involves a one-stage selection process.

- Each participant or object has an equal and independent chance of being drawn.
- The study or accessible population can be identified and listed.

When using this technique, the researcher needs to follow these steps:

1. Define the population.
2. Create a sample frame.
3. Calculate the sample size. This is done using a sampling formula (see statistical textbooks).
4. Assign a consecutive identification number to each element in the sample frame.
5. Select a technique to randomly sample participants.

There are numerous techniques for selecting randomly. The most common entail:

- placing the numbers or names in a bowl or hat and drawing them out one at a time (also known as the 'fishbowl technique')
- using a table of random numbers (see statistical textbooks)
- using a computer-generated selection of random numbers
- using Excel to generate a sample.

Simple random sampling generated using **Excel** will entail the following steps:

1. Write each name or number from the sampling frame, or the list, on a separate slip of paper. For example, if the defined study population consists of all medical doctors in hospital X and there are 100 on the personnel list, the researcher writes out 100 slips. This process can also be followed using online techniques.
2. Put the slips into the bowl or other suitable container. In the case of online selection, the names or numbers are put in a file or cluster.
3. Draw a slip, note the name or number, replace the slip, shake the bowl and select a second, a third, and so on, until the required number is reached according to the sample size calculated. Each slip must be replaced after every selection. This ensures that each participant has an equal, and independent, chance of being selected every time. If this approach is used, each of the 100 names has a 1-in-100 chance of being selected every time. This is called 'random sampling with replacement'. If a participant is selected twice, the researcher should ignore the duplicate and repeat the process until they have the required sample. If 20 names are selected without the slip being returned to the bowl, there would be a 1-in-80 chance of selection. This is called 'random sampling without replacement'.

To use a table of random numbers, the researcher can follow this procedure:

1. Find a table of random numbers (available in most statistical textbooks and online). Tables 10.1 and 10.2 refer. The table is mathematically prepared so that numbers are written in a random manner in rows or columns. The researcher can also generate a table of random numbers using a computer program. This is effective even when large populations are involved.
2. Select a starting point by pointing to a place on the table without looking at it.

3. Beginning with the number selected, choose a direction – that is, horizontal, vertical or diagonal – and continue in a systematic fashion to select the desired number of participants.
4. If a number occurs in a row or column not represented in the population, exclude the number and move to the next.

Table 10.1 Table of random numbers

46	85	04	23	26
69	24	89	34	60
14	01	33	17	92
56	30	38	83	15
81	30	44	85	85

Table 10.2 Sample selected

The researcher needs ten participants randomly selected from a population of individuals numbered from 1 to 80 and arbitrarily begins					
Participants selected are numbers					
33	38	44	23	34	17
73	26	60	15		

In the example above, the population consists of 80 individuals, which implies that two-digit numbers must be selected. The arbitrary starting point is 33. This starting point is selected by blindly placing one's finger or the cursor on some point on the table. The researcher moves down the column and then down the next two until they have selected ten numbers. The researcher must exclude two numbers which are not represented in the population numbers: 85 and 92.

In another example, the researcher must randomly select 40 units out of a population of 400. As 400 consists of three digits, the researcher must select any three adjacent digits and, reading row- or column-wise, write down 40 numbers under the value of 400. Using the random numbers, starting in the top column of the top row and moving along the top row, the first number is 468 whilst the second is 504. Both must be excluded as they are not represented in the population numbers. The first number represented in the population is 232.

A third way of producing a simple random sample also requires that each individual be numbered. Instead of a table of random numbers, a computer-generated set of numbers is used. Usually, more numbers are generated than are expected to constitute the sample because there may be duplications (which will have to be ignored).

Systematic or interval sampling

Systematic sampling involves selecting elements at equal intervals, such as every fifth, eighth or 20th element. This technique is based on the supposition that cases are not added to the list in a systematic way that coincides with the sampling system. If a list of elements or cases is available, systematic sampling is easy and convenient. Moreover, it is often used in clinical practice where, for instance, patients' temperatures and blood pressure are measured every hour.

In systematic sampling, the researcher should follow this procedure:
1. Obtain a list of the total population (N). The elements must be listed randomly. If placed in a specific order (for example, alphabetically, in hierarchical order, or males followed by females), bias may occur because the sample selection cannot be truly representative of the population.
2. Determine the sample size (n).
3. Determine the sampling interval (K) by dividing the size of the population by the sample size.

sampling interval (K)	$\dfrac{\text{size of population}}{\text{size of the sample}}$	$\dfrac{N}{n}$

Figure 10.1 Formula for calculating sampling interval

4. Choose a random starting point – the best way is through a table of random numbers.
5. Select the other elements or units based on the sampling interval. For example, if the population is 400 and the sample size is 80, the sampling interval is 5 (400 ÷ 80). A number between 1 and 400 is randomly selected as the starting number. Imagining that the first randomly selected number is 12, the next four participants will be 17, 22, 27 and 32.

When careful attention is paid to obtaining an unbiased listing of the population elements, and the first element is randomly selected, systematic sampling is classified as probability sampling. If either of the criteria is not met, non-probability sampling occurs.

Stratified random sampling

In stratified random sampling the population is divided into subgroups or strata according to a variable or variables of importance to the study, so that each element of the population belongs to one, and only one, stratum. Then, within each stratum, random sampling is performed, using either the simple or systematic (interval) sampling technique. Various population characteristics may call for the use of stratified sampling. Region (urban, semi-urban and rural), age, gender, educational level and income are examples of variables which may be used as criteria for dividing populations into subgroups. For hospitals, the strata may include criteria like size, public or private, or the number of beds.

For example, the researcher has chosen size as the number of beds in a hospital and is seeking a 50 per cent sample of this group of hospitals. Table 10.3 provides the relevant random sample.

Table 10.3 Example of a random sample stratified according to size

Size	No of hospitals	Proportional sample (50%)
> 1 000	6	3
500–999	8	4
200–499	16	8
200	20	10
	50	25

In Table 10.3 the hospitals are listed in groups according to size. Using a table of random numbers, the researcher draws a 50 per cent sample from each of them. The resulting sample consists of 25 hospitals, with all sizes represented in the same proportion they were in the population. The researcher has therefore selected a proportionate stratified random sample. All segments are proportionately represented in relation to the size of the stratum in the population. This is particularly important when key segments in the population occur in low proportions. Furthermore, the exact representativeness of the sample is known, which has significant statistical value.

Stratified random sampling can also be done using Google Sheets. For more detail, access Google Sheets or watch a YouTube video.

Disproportionate stratified sampling occurs when the number of elements in each stratum is not proportionate to the number in the population. Instead of selecting a 50 per cent sample from each stratum in the above example, the researcher could have selected five hospitals from each group.

The advantage of stratified random sampling is that it provides for the representation of a particular segment of the population. The disadvantages include the following: it requires extensive knowledge of the population in order for it to be stratified, a complete list of the study population is needed, it can be costly, and it can quickly become highly complex.

Cluster sampling

In large-scale studies where the population is geographically widespread, sampling procedures can be difficult and time-consuming. In addition, it may be difficult or even impossible for the researcher to obtain a total listing of some populations. In this case, cluster sampling may be appropriate.

Cluster sampling takes place in stages. The researcher begins with the largest, most inclusive sampling unit and progresses to the next until they reach the final stage – which is the selection of elements or participants in the study. For example, a researcher who wishes to study victims of physical abuse across the country may use regions in South Africa as the largest unit – that is, the nine provinces – then randomly select a sample from the provinces. Next, they identify the hospitals which admit and treat these victims in each of the provinces making up the sample. They select a sample of the hospitals, probably by stratified sampling. The final selection is a sample of victims of physical abuse from the selected sample of hospitals. The clusters considered in this example are thus provinces, hospitals and, finally, patients (victims of physical abuse). The specification of each cluster constitutes a stage, and each stage is characterised by a random sample. Given the successive stages, this technique is often referred to as 'multistage sampling'.

The main advantage of cluster sampling is that it is considerably more economical in terms of time and costs than other techniques of probability sampling, particularly when a population is large and geographically dispersed. There are, however, two major disadvantages:

1. More sampling errors tend to occur than with simple random or stratified random sampling, especially in the first stage.
2. Appropriate handling of statistical data from cluster samples is complex.

Non-probability sampling

Non-probability sampling is widely used in health sciences research. This type of sampling may or may not accurately represent the population. It is usually more convenient and economical and allows for the study of populations when they are not amenable to probability sampling, or when the researcher is unable to locate the entire population. Where access to the participants or elements is limited, the representativeness of the sample also cannot be determined, because it would be impossible for the researcher to specify whether each element has an equal chance of being included in the sample.

Non-probability sampling requires the researcher to assess and select participants who know the most about the phenomenon, and who can articulate and explain nuances. The non-probability sampling plan is constructed from an objective judgement of a likely starting point, and the direction the sampling takes will be a decision made by the researcher as the study progresses (Burns & Grove, 2020; Padgett, 2017). The major techniques of non-probability samples include convenience samples, quota samples, purposive or theoretical samples, and special technique samples such as snowball or network samples.

Non-probability sampling places a greater burden of judgement on the researcher. Its major disadvantages include the following: it does not contribute to generalisation, the extent of sampling error cannot be estimated and bias may be present. Nevertheless, this approach is defensible in many instances. For example, the researcher may not be concerned with the typical experience of the population and is therefore not interested in generalisability. Instead, they may be more concerned with understanding the experience of particular segments of the population or are interested in studying rare or unpredictable phenomena.

The quality of the data obtained from non-probability samples can be high if the researchers have willing participants. The significance of the results has the same potential, depending on the logical and theoretical direction the researcher imposes on the sampling process. Taking care in sample selection, conservatively interpreting results, and replicating the study with new samples mean that the researcher could find that non-probability sampling works well.

In some cases, especially in studies of a clinical nature, the researcher may have to use a non-probability approach if they do not wish to abandon the project. Even uncompromising research consultants would hesitate to advocate the total abandonment of a researcher's ideas in the absence of a random sample.

Online research has become more popular and relevant. Recruiting participants in online research through non-probability sampling could be done in different ways. Although online researchers may still recruit participants face-to-face and in writing, hosting a videoconference has become a good way of reaching the required population. Recruiting participants online could also be done by:

- posting a detailed message with a dedicated email address for responses
- obtaining permission from the host before posting a request for participation in order to respect members' privacy
- initiating discussion on a topic to assess interest
- offering an information session to discuss the proposed study
- communicating individually with all potential participants.

Techniques or types of non-probability sampling

In non-probability sampling, the sampling elements are chosen from the population by non-random methods.

Convenience sampling

Convenience sampling is also referred to as 'accidental' or 'availability' sampling and involves the choice of readily available participants or objects for the study. It is generally considered a poor sampling type because it provides little opportunity to control bias. Elements are included in the sample because they happen to be in the right place at the right time. The researcher may choose, for example, the first 25 homeless people visiting a soup kitchen for an interview, or the patients available in a specific ward on a certain day. This can introduce certain biases as some elements may be over-

or under-represented. Generalisation based on such samples is precarious, though, despite the samples being convenient for researchers in terms of time and costs. While it is used in studies where probability sampling is not possible, this type of sampling should be used only when samples are unobtainable or difficult to reach by other means, especially in quantitative studies. This technique is, however, often used in qualitative research where the intention is not to generalise the findings.

Quota sampling

This sampling technique could be considered the non-probability equivalent of stratified sampling. Its purpose is to draw a sample with the same proportions or characteristics as the entire population. However, instead of relying on random choice, the sampling procedure relies on convenience choice. The aim of quota sampling is to replicate the proportions of subgroups or strata present in the population.

The researcher first determines which strata are to be studied. Common strata are age groups, gender, race, geographic locations and socio-economic groups. The researcher then determines a quota, or number, of participants needed for each stratum. Procedurally, quota sampling is like convenience sampling as the participants are a convenience sample from each stratum. The quota may be determined proportionately or disproportionately.

For a proportionate quota sample, the researcher must obtain information on the population's composition. If the population consists of 60 per cent women, the sample should also consist of 60 per cent men. The ratio is thus the same. For example, the population under study is estimated to consist of 40 per cent men and 60 per cent women. Twenty-five per cent of the men are older than 40 and 15 per cent are between 20 and 40 years of age. Of the 60 per cent women, 30 per cent are in each of these age groups. If the researcher intends to draw a sample of 200, they interview people in each stratum 'as they come', that is, using convenience sampling, until they have gathered 80 men (40 per cent of 200), of whom 50 are older than 40 and 30 are between 20 and 40 years of age. The female subsample consists of 120 women, with 60 in each age category. Disproportionate sampling would occur, for example, if the researcher decided to use 50 per cent males and 50 per cent females and 25 per cent from each of the age groups.

Purposive/judgemental sampling

Purposive sampling is sometimes also called 'judgemental' sampling and is another type of non-probability sampling. This technique is thus based on the researcher's judgement regarding participants or objects that are typical, or representative, of the study phenomenon, or who are especially knowledgeable. Alternatively, the researcher may wish to interview individuals who reflect different ends of a characteristic's range: for example, a comparison between patients who display a low pain threshold and those who experience a high pain threshold. In a more complex example a researcher who wants to investigate attitudes towards death in HIV-positive individuals may select participants who do not yet display symptoms and those who have active disease symptoms and are considered terminal.

Purposive sampling is commonly seen in qualitative research. This sampling technique requires the judgement of the researcher and may lead to bias although it is a useful approach when the researcher wants a sample of experts. As the qualitative researcher using this method does not know in advance how many participants are needed, they sample continuously until data saturation (the point at which new data no longer emerge during the data-collection process) occurs. No new information is achieved, and redundancy is achieved, leaving the researcher with a sense of closure. The number of participants needed to reach data saturation will differ from study to study as it will depend on various factors. The scope of the study, knowledgeability and insightfulness of participants on the phenomenon under investigation, and the ability to communicate freely and effectively, are all aspects affecting the stage of data saturation.

The advantage of purposive sampling is that it allows the researcher to select the sample based on knowledge of the phenomena being studied. The disadvantages are the potential for sampling bias, the use of a sample that does not represent the population, and the limited generalisability of the results.

Padgett (2017) describes various types of purposive sampling, namely extreme or deviant case sampling, intensity sampling, maximum variation sampling, homogeneous sampling, typical case sampling, critical case sampling and criterion sampling.

Theoretical sampling

'Theoretical sampling' is the term applied to a more elaborate process used in conjunction with the analysis of data in grounded theory, with a focus on theory development. Theoretical sampling in grounded theory means that the researcher needs specific data to develop the emerging theory and to refine the categories until no new properties emerge (Charmaz, 2014). The researcher collects data from any person or group able to provide relevant, varied and detailed information of theory generation. Data are considered relevant and detailed if they include information that generates, delimits and saturates the theoretical codes in the study needed for theory generation. As the analysis reveals the relationships between the elements of the emerging theory, new sample participants are sought to clarify, extend and refute the findings (Creswell, 2013).

Snowball sampling

Snowball sampling involves the assistance of study participants in obtaining other participants, especially where it is difficult for the researcher to gain access to the population. This type of sampling consists of different stages. First, the researcher identifies a few people with the required characteristics. They then aid the researcher to identify more people who also possess the desired characteristics and who are included in the next stage. The process continues until the researcher is satisfied that the sample is sufficiently large. For example, the researcher wants to determine how to help homeless people to receive primary healthcare services and may know of a homeless person who attends the primary healthcare clinic in his area. The researcher then contacts him to find out whether he knows of others who have also attended the primary healthcare clinic. This type of networking is particularly useful for finding people who are reluctant to make their identity known.

Consecutive sampling

Consecutive sampling involves recruiting all individuals or elements from the accessible population for a specific sample size or of a particular time interval period. This sampling technique is useful where there is a 'rolling' enrollment (Polit & Beck, 2022: 143). For example, in a study of Covid-19-related depression in a mental health institution, a consecutive sample may consist of all eligible patients admitted to the institution over a period of one year. The research may also decide to include the first 30 eligible patients based on the specific sample size decided upon.

Sample choice

The choice of sample is closely related to the study design. For example, a researcher studying an area in which little knowledge has accumulated would select a level 1 question and a qualitative design. A probability sample would not be suitable. If, however, the researcher seeks to test hypotheses, a non-probability sample would be unsuitable. The suitability of a sampling type for a particular design type could be controversial in instances where there is an overlap between the types of design suited to a study. In mixed methods research the sample choice will be guided by the type of design used and based on each phase of the study. A blend of approaches is therefore used. A unique sampling issue of mixed methods research is where the same individuals will be used in both the qualitative and quantitative phases. Although the purpose of the study and the research design will determine the sample selection, there could be an advantage of using overlapping samples. This is referred to as a 'nested' approach, where a subset of the study participants from the quantitative phase is used in the qualitative phase.

The sample choice is based on a critical appraisal of the sampling plan. The researcher's decision is based on the:

- type of sampling approach suitable for the study
- type of sampling technique selected
- population and eligibility criteria
- sample size and the rationale for it
- main characteristics of the participants (clinical status, age, knowledge about the phenomenon).

Sample size

Sample size differs in quantitative research and qualitative research. Selecting and obtaining the appropriate sample size are problems every researcher faces. While there are no precise rules that can be applied to the determination of sample size, the researcher must consider both scientific and pragmatic factors influencing it when they decide on the number of participants to be included in a study. These factors vary according to the purpose, design and type of sample used. Therefore, sample size cannot be transferred from one study to another and must be calculated anew for each research problem.

It is a misconception that the larger the sample, the better it is. While a large sample can be advantageous in quantitative studies, this holds true only up to a point, and is not applicable to qualitative studies. Grove, Gray and Burns (2015) and Polit and Beck (2021) suggest that as the population increases in size, the sample size required for precision in estimation remains constant, and that the absolute size of the sample is more important than the sample size relative to population size. However, as sample size increases, sampling error decreases. Furthermore, with regard to a probability sample and the precision of how closely the sample value relates to the population value, Bryman (2008: 179) suggests that 'equal precision' is found in the following samples:

- When the population is 2 000 and the sample is 200 (10 per cent of the population).
- When the population is 100 000 and the sample is 200 (2 per cent of the population).

Roestenburg et al (2021) suggest that a study with an over-large sample may be deemed unnecessary. A large sample is no guarantee of accuracy, and one with a poor design can inflate error and bias. Indeed, because of the involvement of extra participants and the correspondingly increased costs, this kind of study can become unethical. Similarly, a study with a sample that is too small may not be able to detect clinically important effects.

When using probability sampling in quantitative studies, the researcher can calculate the exact number of participants needed according to how much sampling error they are willing to accept. Various statistical textbooks (Ader & Mellenbergh, 1999; Polgar & Thomas, 2000) provide formulae for calculating the effect of size, and tables for many types of statistical tests that show the required sample size. You can also find a variety of electronic options for calculating sample size, such as the 'sample size calculator' at http://www. surveysystem.com/sscalc.htm or https://www.macorr.com/sample-size-calculator.htm.

In qualitative studies, where the type of sample is usually purposive, too many participants would increase the complexity of the analysis process. For these types of studies, the sample size is adequate when the meanings are clear and data are fully explored (Breakwell, Hammond & Fife-Schaw, 2000; Polit & Beck, 2021). The trend, however, indicates a shift away from samples that are too small to numbers of 20 or even 30 or more in qualitative studies. Sample sizes smaller than this imply that the findings may be idiosyncratic and make it easier for the researcher to observe the identity of the participants. Nevertheless, it is important that data saturation occurs and that each qualitative study's sample size is guided by addressing the research question. Data saturation happens when additional sampling yields no new information, and only redundancy of data already collected (Gray, Grove & Sutherland, 2017; LoBiondo-Wood & Haber, 2014).

Table 10.4 summarises the factors that the researcher should consider when choosing a sample size.

Table 10.4 Factors influencing the choice of sample size

Factor	Things to remember and consider
Accuracy needed	As the sample size increases, so too does the accuracy (to a point)
Population size	As the size of the population increases, a smaller proportion of participants can be selected Survey designs usually require large numbers of participants
Nature of research design	Qualitative studies are conducted with fewer participants
Type of research	Preferably a minimum of 30 participants is needed per variable or phenomenon
Heterogeneity	The sample size must grow as the number of variables increases – more participants are needed
Methods of data collection	If methods are not precise, a larger sample is required
Research hypothesis	Where slight differences are expected, a larger sample is required
Statistical analyses to be used	Sample size can be expressed as the value of the indicators
Financial resources	Must relate to the availability of resources
Attrition rate	Often expected, may influence sample size

Besides the nature of the design and the degree of accuracy required, several other factors should be considered in determining sample size. These include:

- **Precision of the data-collection instrument.** A study which uses a crude measure will generally have to sample more participants to obtain a reasonable estimate of population parameters than one where the data-collection instrument is more precise. The less precise the tool, the larger the sample needed.

- **Heterogeneity of the population.** As the number of demographic variables increases, so must the sample size. Most researchers agree that there should be at least ten participants for each variable, with 20 to 30 preferred.
- **Incidence of participant type in the population.** Greater numbers of participants are required in cases where the incidence of the study phenomenon is rare. Statistical analyses also impose certain requirements regarding sample size.

Sampling is an integral part of the research process and should not be considered in isolation. When planning samples, the researcher should consider the sample in relation to the research question, purpose and design, as well as practical reality. This is beneficial because it reduces the time and costs that the researcher needs to complete the study.

Sample adequacy

It is important that both the researcher and the research consumer evaluate the adequacy of the sample. Several aspects of the sampling procedure must be systematically evaluated. A checklist is presented below.

- Are the target population, accessible population and sample described?
- Was a probability or non-probability sampling approach used?
- Is/are the specific sampling technique(s) named and described?
- Does the sample type fit with the design type?
- Does the sample type fit with the study's purpose?
- If a non-probability sampling approach is used, how is representativeness accounted for?
- Is a methodological or theoretical rationale for the sample size clearly explained?
- Is the sample size similar to those in comparable studies?
- For qualitative studies, is there an adequate number of participants to describe the phenomenon, but not so many as to cloud the issues surrounding it?
- For studies with a probability sample, was a power analysis done?
- Are inclusion/eligibility or exclusion (where applicable) criteria listed?
- Is any participant attrition (or participant drop-out) clearly described?
- Are biases reflected in the interpretation of the results?
- Have sources of sampling error been controlled or minimised?
- Is enough information given so that another researcher would be able to replicate the sampling procedures?

Summary

In this chapter, we paid attention to the various aspects of sampling, and explained the basic sampling concepts. We described the two major approaches to sampling, as well as the common techniques or types. The chapter closed by exploring sample size and giving guidelines for evaluating the adequacy of a sample.

Exercises

1. What is the rationale behind the use of samples? Should samples be used only when a complete list of a population is unavailable? Give reasons for your answer.

2. You would like to study the effects of music on ventilated patients.

   (a) What would your target population be?

   (b) What would your accessible population be?

   (c) What are your inclusion (or eligibility) criteria?

3. Using the table of random numbers provided in Table 10.1, draw a sample of five units out of a population of 270.

4. Formulate a research question for an online quantitative study. Plan your sampling technique for this study.

5. Using the same example as in question 4, justify your sampling choice.

6. Argue the value of purposive sampling in qualitative research.

7. Explain the concept of data saturation. What would make you decide that data saturation was reached after 15 interviews?

8. Select an article from a research journal. Evaluate the sampling section of the research report.

9. Using the same example as in question 8, propose and justify a different sampling approach or technique.

Data collection

This chapter focuses on the data-collection methods, procedures and techniques planned as part of the research design. Data collection aims to address the research question and is critically important to a study's success. Without quality data-collection techniques, the accuracy of the research is easily challenged. It is therefore essential that the researcher is familiar with the various techniques, including their advantages and disadvantages, so that they can select the one most suitable for the study purpose, setting and population.

The data-collection process

Data collection describes the way in which the researcher approaches answering the research question (Maree, 2016). This process is a research component (step in the research process) in all study fields, be it human and social sciences, natural sciences, literature reviews or creative arts research. It provides an audit trail which includes a clear and specific explanation of how data were collected, how the results or findings were derived, and the rationale for the method selected.

When planning the data collection process, the researcher is guided by five important questions:

1. What data do I want to collect?
2. How will it be collected?
3. Who will collect the data?
4. Where will it be collected?
5. When will the data be collected?

What data will be collected?

The researcher must carefully consider what information is needed to answer the research question. For example, does the question call for knowledge, or attitudes or behaviours? If the researcher is concerned with the way in which the Covid-19 pandemic affected the use of healthcare services, the what of data collection becomes healthcare users' behaviours, experiences or responses during a disruptive period/pandemic. The researcher must also consider whether to quantify the data or analyse it qualitatively. In the former case a decision must be made regarding the level of measurement, or the measurement scale to be used. In the latter case the researcher would be interested in the narrated responses and in what form they will be collected, such as interviews, reflective journals or data in the form of visual presentation (e g drawings).

Nominal scales

The lowest category of measurement is the nominal scale measurement and is used when data can be organised into specific categories of a defined property. These categories cannot be ranked. Therefore, nominal scales are used when persons, events or other phenomena are separated into mutually exclusive categories: for example, married or single, divorced or widowed, dead or alive. At this level of measurement, the categories cannot be ordered as being 'more than', 'higher than' or 'larger than'. The nominal scales are thus exclusive and exhaustive categories.

Ordinal scales

Ordinal scales are used for variables that can be categorised and rank ordered or assessed incrementally, therefore being higher or lower, or better or worse than another category. Like nominal data, the categories must be exclusive where each datum fits into only one category. These categories can be ranked, meaning the quantity can be identified. A typical example is the different categories to measure the intensity and levels of pain. The categories could be unbearable, severe, moderate, mild and no pain. In this example you may be able to identify the level of pain but not the intervals between the levels of pain. Therefore, the pain may move fast from unbearable to severe but slow from severe to moderate. You therefore cannot know with certainty that the intervals between the ranked categories are equal. Another example of ordinal measurement could be the feelings of a person's happiness being classified not only as happy or sad, but also more specifically as extremely happy, happy, indifferent, unhappy or extremely unhappy, thus enabling the comparison between degrees of a person's happiness. Other examples of ordinal scales are when the categories are ranked from 0 to 5: 0 = no oedema of feet; 1 = minimal oedema of feet; 2 = moderate oedema of feet; 3 = extreme oedema of feet; and 4 = oedema so severe that patient is unable to walk without assistance. In the latter case the researcher could conclude that extreme oedema is greater than moderate oedema, but they cannot determine the exact difference in oedema between moderate and intense as oedema cannot be directly measured. The ordinal scales are thus exclusive, exhaustive and ranked categories.

Interval scales

Variables within the interval scale of measurement are assigned real numbers which are categorised and ordered with equal measurement between each category. The categories in interval data are the actual numbers on a scale, like those on a thermometer. If body temperature is being measured, a reading of 36.2 °C could be one category, 37.0 °C another and 37.8 °C a third. The researcher would conclude that there is a difference of 0.8 °C between the first and second categories, as well as between the second and third – indicating equal intervals. Similarly, if the researcher undertakes a study in which a psychological test is used, the scores will represent interval data. Two hundred people completed the test and 90 obtained scores between 40 and 49, 30 obtained scores between 50 and 59, 60 obtained scores between 60 and 69, and 20 obtained scores between 70 and 79. The scores are categorised into interval classes, which means that they are ranked and the measurements between each class are equal. The rule of mutually exclusive, exhaustive and ranked categories with a continuum of values with equal intervals applies in this form of measurement.

Ratio scales

Ratio-level measurement is the highest form of measurement. A ratio level of measurement includes data which can be categorised and ranked. The difference between ranks can be specified and a true (or natural) zero point can be identified. The number of tablets in a bottle, for example, could be considered ratio data because it is possible for it to be zero. In the case of the number of pain medication requests made by two groups of patients, it is possible that some patients in one group do not ask for medication. This type of data would be considered ratio data. Other obvious ratio scales include time, length and weight. The rule of mutually exclusive, exhaustive and ranked categories with a continuum of values with an absolute zero and equal intervals applies in this form of measurement.

If a researcher designs a qualitative study, they are not concerned with measurement scales and collect data in narrative form instead. The type of data needed also governs the how, who, where and when of the data-collection process. The answers to these questions are interrelated. The four measurement scales are discussed further in Chapter 13.

How will data be collected?

The researcher must use an instrument to gather the data. The type can vary from a checklist to a questionnaire to a sophisticated physiological measure. The choice of instrument is a decision that should be made only after careful consideration of the topic under investigation, the research question and the context. It is also important that the manner in which data are captured is reliable. For example, if audio recorders are used, the researcher should ensure that these are in working order, and that fieldworkers know how to use them. In online data collection the security of the software programs must be considered. Raw data needs to be stored in a safe place, ensuring security, especially if it has not yet been anonymised.

Who will collect the data?

Data collection could be done by one researcher, such as in a degree research project, or in teams of various sizes. A researcher may appoint a fieldworker to assist with data collection. In collaborative research the team may consist of a number of researchers and fieldworkers. Data collectors can be paid for their services. However, it is necessary to ensure that data are gathered in the same manner whenever more than one person is involved. In addition, where fieldworkers are used as data collectors, they need training, and the reliability of the collected data must be checked.

Where will the data be collected?

The setting for data collection must be carefully determined. It could take place in a controlled laboratory, a classroom, a ward, a clinic, a home, a community centre, within a specific region, and so on.

When will the data be collected?

The researcher must decide exactly when data are to be collected, as well as how long the process will last. The researcher must carefully consider aspects such as time of day, circumstances such as waiting in a queue to see a doctor, and active patient care time. It is important that the data collection does not take place when, for example, it may influence quality of care, patients' rights or teaching time. Sometimes the only way to answer this question is by conducting a trial or pilot study to get a good understanding of the context within which the data collection will take place.

Data-collection methods

There are various data-collection methods. The ones used most frequently by healthcare professionals include observation, self-report and physiological methods.

Observation

Observation is a method used for collecting **descriptive** data on behaviour, events and situations. It is useful in health sciences context because it allows the researcher to observe behaviour as it occurs. To be considered scientific, observation must be made under precisely defined conditions in a systematic and objective manner, with careful record-keeping. All observations must be checked and controlled. These criteria transform the simple act of observing the world into a purposeful act of collecting data.

Observations may be structured or unstructured. **Structured observations** entail specifying in advance the behaviours or events to be observed and how they will be recorded, as well as preparing forms (such as checklists, categorisation systems and rating scales) for record-keeping. Structured observation is commonly used in quantitative studies, where the researcher or fieldworker (trained observer) observes and records certain aspects of participants' behaviour – examples being healthcare professionals' willingness to interact with, and listen to, patients; the interaction between a mother and her newborn baby; two students engaging in a simulated nurse–patient consultation; verbal communication behaviours when handing over the patient report; patients' eating habits; and children's reactions to the removal of a plaster cast from one of their legs or arms. In the last example, behaviours to be observed may be nurse–patient interaction, distress in a child, co-operation and a need for information. The researcher could prepare a rating scale which provides a score on these behaviours and record on the scale what they observe. Structured observation requires knowledge about the expected range of behaviours in each scenario. When developing a checklist, for instance, the researcher must list all expected behaviours related to the variable being measured.

Unstructured observation involves the collection of descriptive information which is analysed qualitatively rather than quantitatively. In unstructured observations the researcher attempts to describe events or behaviours as they occur, with no pre-conceived ideas of what they will see or pre-set criteria and categories. For example, an unstructured observation method may be used to describe the behaviour of a nurse immediately following the death of one of their patients. It would involve a complete description of everything the nurse says and does at this time. Observations could be recorded by video after which careful observations could be made and detailed notes could be taken at a later stage. Common forms of record-keeping include logs and field notes. A log is a daily record of events and conversations that have taken place, while field notes may include the daily log, but tend to encompass more than a simple list of occurrences. It will include non-verbal cues such as facial expressions, tone of voice and bodily movements (such as fiddling).

Observations can also be categorised according to the degree of researcher involvement. Polit and Beck (2021) mention various levels of participation during observation.

Timing of observations

Since it is not possible for the researcher to observe behaviours for extended periods of time, it is necessary for them to plan when, and how, to make observations. The examples which follow involve nurse–patient interaction. The two primary methods are time sampling and event sampling. **Time sampling** involves observing events during specified times: for example, to observe nurse–patient interaction, several 15-minute periods during an eight-hour shift would provide a good sample of interactions. The periods can be either randomly selected or predetermined according to the daily routine of the ward.

Event sampling involves observing an entire event, ie if a researcher is interested in determining nurse–patient interaction during admission to hospital, event sampling would be appropriate because the researcher would observe the entire admission procedure. In this case they must either have some knowledge concerning the occurrence of events or be able to wait for that occurrence.

Advantages and disadvantages of observation

Scientific observation has several advantages as a data-collection method. Many healthcare problems are better suited to an observational approach than to questionnaires or interviews. Examples of situations where observation is suitable are the manifestation of pre-operative signs of anxiety, displays of aggression or hostility. No other data-collection method matches the depth and variety of information which can be collected through observational techniques. These techniques are also flexible and can be used in both experimental and non-experimental designs, as well as in laboratory and field studies.

Disadvantages include problems concerning the reactions of the observed when they are aware that they are being observed. Ethical issues may arise if the researcher does not obtain consent, as data obtained through observation are vulnerable to bias and distortion. Emotions, prejudices and values can all influence the way in which behaviours and events are observed. Observation is also time-consuming and can be costly, particularly when the observers must undergo training.

Guidelines for critiquing observational methods

The following questions should be considered when observation has been used:

- Is observation an appropriate approach to obtain the necessary information?
- What, or who, must be observed?
- Was a structured or unstructured approach used, and to what extent was the researcher involved?
- Did the researcher explain where and when the observations occurred?
- Was the time of the observation appropriate to addressing the research question?
- Was the location where the observation was done appropriate to addressing the research question?
- Was the length of time spent to observe the situation recorded?
- Was the time adequate to collect comprehensive and exhaustive data?
- Did the researcher explain how the data were recorded?
- Were fieldnotes made during the observation?
- What steps were taken to minimise observer bias?

Self-report techniques

When the researcher's objective is to find out what people believe, think or know, the easiest and most effective method is to direct the questions to them. In addition to gathering factual information about the participants, the purpose of questions is to discover their thoughts, perceptions, attitudes, beliefs, feelings, motives, plans, experiences, knowledge levels and memories. Since participants must answer the questions about the study variable directly, these techniques are known as 'self-report' techniques, and self-report instruments include questionnaires, scales and interviews.

The type of self-report instrument chosen depends on the research objectives and sample. Verbal techniques such as interviews (individual and focus group), and written techniques such as questionnaires and scales, have varying strengths and weaknesses. The researcher must consider these aspects when choosing the instrument. Table 11.1 presents the strengths and weaknesses of interviews and questionnaires.

Questionnaires

In the questionnaire process the respondent, who is the unit of analysis, writes down their answers in response to questions in a printed or online document. A well-designed questionnaire is easy for the respondent to complete if they are literate and is also easy for the researcher to administer and score. Questionnaires are, however, difficult to develop. Each aspect – from the questions themselves to the colour of the print or paper or lay-out of the online questionnaire – can influence respondents' replies. The researcher must therefore pay careful attention to the development and construction of the questionnaire.

A well-designed questionnaire should:

- meet the objectives of the inquiry
- demonstrate a fit between its contents and the research problem and objectives
- obtain the most complete, accurate information possible, and do so within reasonable limits of time and resources.

Table 11.1 Strengths and weaknesses of interviews and questionnaires

Interviews	Questionnaires
Strengths	
1. The participant need not be able to read or write 2. Responses can be obtained from a wide range of participants – almost all segments of the population 3. Responses and retention role are high 4. Non-verbal behaviour and mannerisms can bo oboorvcd 5. Questions may be clarified if they are misunderstood 6. In-depth responses can be obtained	1. Questionnaires are a quick way of obtaining data from a large group of people 2. They are less expensive in terms of time and money 3. They are one of the easiest research instruments for testing reliability and validity 4. Participants feel a greater sense of anonymity, and are more likely to provide honest answers 5. There is a standard format for all participants

Weaknesses	
1. Training programmes are needed for interviewers	1. Mailing questionnaires may be expensive
2. Interviews can be time-consuming and expensive	2. Response rate may be low
3. Arranging interviews may be difficult	3. Respondents may provide socially acceptable answers
4. Participants may provide socially acceptable responses	4. Respondents may fail to answer some of the questions
5. Participants may be anxious because answers are being recorded	5. There is no opportunity to clarify questions which may be misunderstood by participants
6. Participants may be influenced by interviewer characteristics	6. Participants must be literate
7. Interviewers may misinterpret non-verbal behaviour	7. The participants who respond may not be representative of the population

When developing a questionnaire, bear these important points in mind:

- List the specific research issues to be investigated by the questionnaire. Clearly specified goals and objectives, research questions and/or unambiguous hypotheses are significant precursors to asking the right questions.
- Ensure you have a thorough understanding of the relevant literature.
- Analyse the kind of information needed for the research questions.
- Formulate specific questions and test each for precision of expression, relevance, objectivity, suitability, and the probability of reception and return (Leedy & Ormrod, 2010).

Using a specification matrix with the various content areas in which questions covering specific situations are needed is helpful. Once the areas are identified, the researcher can decide what proportion of questioning time to allocate to each. For example, if you are interested in the attitudes towards the use of restraints with regard to hospitalised geriatric patients, the specification matrix may resemble that provided in Figure 11.1. This matrix directs you to develop ten questions for each cell for a total questionnaire length of 40 questions. This relatively simple matrix indicates that the researcher considers all elements to be equally important.

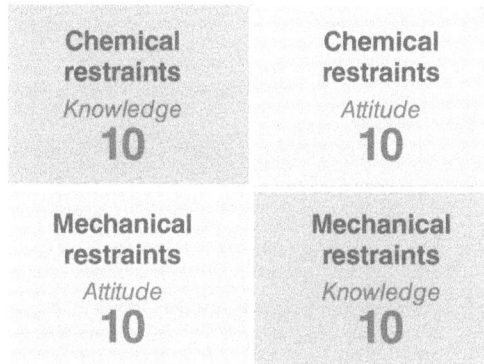

| Chemical restraints *Knowledge* **10** | Chemical restraints *Attitude* **10** |
| Mechanical restraints *Attitude* **10** | Mechanical restraints *Knowledge* **10** |

Figure 11.1 An example of a specification matrix

In order to obtain a certain type of answer the researcher needs to consider the construction of their questions. They may seek a long, detailed answer which reflects the individuality of the respondents, or a short one selected from the categories provided. The researcher thus must choose between using unstructured, open-ended questions or structured, closed-ended ones. The former allow the respondent to answer in any way they see fit, while the latter require the respondent to choose from a set of options. Closed-ended questions can be 'yes' or 'no', multiple-choice, checklist-type, 'true' or 'false', and matching questions.

Examples of open-ended questions include:
- How would you describe the general views of the community about the proposed National Health Insurance plan?
- What are your views on using cannabis for pain relief in cancer patients?

Table 11.2 provides examples of closed-ended questions.

Table 11.2 Closed-ended questions

Question type	Example
Dichotomous question	Have you very been for surgery? 1. Yes 2. No
Multiple choice question	How scared are you to go for surgery for the first time? 1. Extremely scared 2. Very scared 3. Neutral 4. Somewhat scared 5. Not scared

Question type	Example
Forced-choice question	Which statement mostly describes your anxiety about having surgery? 1. I do not have enough information on the surgical procedure to be anxious about it. 2. I am anxious about the surgery because I know I will have pain afterwards.
Rating questions	On a scale of 1–10, where 0 means not anxious at all, and 10 means extremely anxious, how anxious are you about having surgery?

A structured, closed-ended alternative to an open-ended question such as 'What led you to use cannabis as pain relief alternative?' could be 'Was your decision to use cannabis as a pain relief alternative mainly determined by:

- your fear of Western medicine
- your social environment
- your interest in holistic medicine
- the unavailability of effective pain medication?'

Open-ended questions are not based on preconceived answers and are appropriate for exploratory studies, case studies or studies based on qualitative analyses of data. They generally provide richer, more diverse data than can be obtained with the use of closed-ended questions. These questions are easier to construct, although they take longer to answer, and the very diversity of the answers makes them more difficult for the researcher to code and analyse. Issues of validity and reliability also come to the fore.

Closed-ended questions limit the answers to options provided by the researcher. The greater the complexity of the mental tasks that respondents are required to perform, the more other answering aids (such as visual aids) help to obtain true answers. This has several advantages for the researcher. It facilitates the coding and analysis of data. Respondents are able to complete more closed-ended questions in a given amount of time and are often more willing to complete closed-ended questions. A drawback of closed-ended questions, though, is that they are more difficult to construct, and it is possible for the researcher to neglect or overlook potentially significant responses. Closed-ended questions may also be superficial, and some respondents can become frustrated with the limited responses provided and the response options that are specified.

Important guidelines to attend to when formulating questions are the following:
- The questions should be **simple** and **short**. Complex questions should be broken up into several simpler ones.
- Questions should not be 'double-barrelled', that is, contain two questions. For

example: 'Do you plan to pursue a Master's degree in your clinical speciality and seek an administrative position upon graduation?' This question should be divided into two separate questions.

- Questions should be **unambiguous**. Words which are too general or vague, or that could be misinterpreted, should be replaced with more specific terms. For instance, words like 'sometimes', 'often', 'many' and 'enough' should be replaced by 'three times a week', 'twelve', 'three meals a day', and so on.
- Questions should be **understandable**. Vocabulary adapted to the participants' level of education should be used. Jargon and sophisticated language should be avoided. Carefully consider the level of education, reading level and potential language barriers that may be characteristic of the respondents when constructing the question.
- **Leading** questions – questions that favour one type of answer over another – should be avoided. For example, 'Don't you agree that . . .?' and '. . . is it not so?'
- Questions should be stated in an **affirmative** manner. For example, 'students are accompanied by a clinical facilitator in the clinical practice daily'. The options would then be 'yes' or 'no'. Rather than: 'Students are not accompanied by a clinical facilitator in the clinical practice daily'.

The arrangement of questions in a questionnaire is critical. They must be arranged in a way that is logical and relevant to the respondent. There are various strategies which can help:

- Start with a covering letter. This is the study's information leaflet and should include an explanation of how the ethical issues will be dealt with. The covering letter may be the single most important factor in motivating respondents. When writing the covering letter, you should try to imagine yourself as the recipient. Clear, comprehensive and concise instructions should also be submitted with the questionnaire, and it is helpful to provide respondents with an example of the appropriate way to respond to particular types of questions.
- Group together similar questions, or all questions about a certain topic. You would typically start with the questions on demographic data. The objectives of the study could also guide the logical flow of the questionnaire. For example, if you are studying the knowledge of students on diabetes, you should group questions about causes of diabetes in one section and those concerning treatment in another.
- The order of questions must be psychologically meaningful to encourage co-operation and openness.
- Ask interesting and/or easier questions first.
- Ask for sensitive information last. Respondents are more likely to answer sensitive questions when they are placed at the end of the questionnaire.
- Arrange questions from general topics to specific ones.
- Repeat the content of a question, formulated in different ways, in different parts of the questionnaire. This is a method of checking the truthfulness of the answers (or the honesty of the respondent) and is useful for topics about which the respondent may have reason to be untruthful.

The questionnaire should be long enough to obtain all the necessary information, but not so long that it tires or bores the respondent. It is recommended that questionnaires take no more than 20 to 25 minutes to complete. However, the length may vary according to the depth of the study. Indicate beforehand what the time expectancy by approximation will be. A long questionnaire may discourage responses, increase non-response or withdrawal from the study, and can prove costly.

Once the questionnaire has been drafted, it should be critically reviewed by others knowledgeable about instrument construction and the content, as well as by a non-specialist who can give insight based on their knowledge of the topic and the sample. The instrument should also be pre-tested with a small sample of respondents and revised if necessary. A pre-test determines whether the instrument is clearly worded and free from major biases, as well as if it is appropriate for the type of information. Other problems could be identified such as the level of sensitivity of the questions and omitted information.

A questionnaire should be neat in appearance and grammatically correct, with no typing or spelling errors, in order to motivate the respondent to address the questions. It should not be cluttered: questions should be well spaced and surrounded by adequate margins. Electronically generated questionnaires must have clear instruction on how to proceed from one question to the next.

There are many methods of distributing questionnaires: they can be emailed as attachments or with a direct link to the online questionnaire, hand-delivered, given in groups, or administered one-on-one.

Questionnaires via electronic means

Collecting data through online surveys has become quite popular. The researcher can develop the questionnaire in a word processing program and distribute it via email. The completed questionnaire is then emailed back or directly delivered to a specific email address once the submit button is pressed. Alternatively, respondents may decide to print the questionnaire and post or fax it back.

Web-based surveys are inexpensive and can reach a large population. They are often less time-consuming and are aligned with the latest communication trends – a motivator for some respondents. However, Polit and Beck (2021) point out that the response rate in such a survey could be lower than in other more traditional survey methods. Some of the reasons are an overload of invitations to participate in a variety of studies, email congestion and the length of the questionnaire.

A website on which the survey will be placed is required, or the researcher can make use of services such as SurveyMonkey or Qualtrics. Respondents are provided with a hyperlink they can use to complete the questionnaire and have the opportunity to receive, as well as give, information.

The researcher may use both methods of distribution, hand-delivered and electronic, in instances where one method does not yield enough responses. Where some respondents have access to email and others do not, it would also be wise to use both means.

Interviews

Interviews obtain responses from participants in face-to-face encounters, through a telephonic conversation, or by electronic means such as Teams, Zoom or Webex. Interviews are frequently used in exploratory and descriptive research, and in case studies. They are the most direct method of obtaining facts from interviewees and can be useful in ascertaining values, preferences, interests, tasks, attitudes, beliefs and experience.

Data-collection interviews are generally classified as either structured or unstructured. Most interviews, however, range between the two, and are thus referred to as 'semi-structured'.

Structured interviews are formalised so that all interviewees hear the same questions in the same order and in the same manner. These interviews are most appropriate when straightforward, factual information is desired. The instrument used here is the interview schedule. The interview schedule uses closed-ended or fixed alternative questions, as well as indications of how the interviewee should answer. It must be presented to each interviewee in exactly the same way. The interviewer is restricted to the questions provided and must ask them in the order in which they appear. There is therefore, relatively little freedom for deviation – this is done to minimise the role and influence of the interviewer and to enable a more objective comparison of results.

The **unstructured interview's** structure is limited only by the research focus. It leaves the wording and organisation of questions, and sometimes even the topic, to the interviewer's discretion. The interviews are conducted in a conversational manner, but with purpose. They are particularly useful for exploratory or qualitative research studies, where the researcher cannot structure questions before data collection takes place. The interviewer may begin with a broad opening question like: 'How do you feel about caring for patients who are crime offenders?' Depending on the interviewee's replies, the researcher invites them to add information or to clarify the initial response.

Probe follow-ups can be used to increase detailed exploration. Probes are prompting questions which encourage the interviewee to elaborate. For example, 'Tell me more about ...', 'What do you mean by ...?', 'Could you please describe ...?', 'I am not sure I understand. Could you explain further?' and 'How did you feel then?' Such follow up questions give the interviewer an opportunity to clarify and expand responses and explicate meaning. They also enhance rapport between interviewer and interviewee. Unstructured interviews will produce in-depth information regarding the interviewees' beliefs and attitudes that cannot be obtained through any other data-gathering procedure.

Semi-structured interviews usually fall somewhere between the structured and unstructured interviews. During a semi-structured interview, the interviewer must ask a specified number of questions, but can also pose additional ones. Both closed-ended and open-ended questions are included in semi-structured interviews.

Focus group interviews include groups of about five to twelve people whose opinions and experiences are requested simultaneously. Grove, Gray and Burns (2015) indicate that the ideal size for a focus group is five to eight participants, Stewart and Shamdasani (2015) posit that eight to twelve participants form the ideal, while Padgett (2017) maintains that although five to seven participants is ideal, as few as three could also suffice (provided enough diversity in opinions can be generated). The researcher must carefully consider the size of the focus group when planning the study and could be guided by the topic, its sensitivity and the type of participants to be included.

Apart from the practical advantages, this method allows participants to share their thoughts with one another, generate new ideas and consider a range of views before answering. Focus groups are particularly useful in participatory and action research where members of the community are equal participants in planning and implementation, and where the topic implies a practical community concern. A disadvantage, however, is that some people are uncomfortable when asked to participate in group discussions. The researcher should thus be skilled at facilitating them. Involving a co-facilitator in focus group interviews must be decided upon carefully. The presence of a second person may limit openness during the discussions, especially where the participants have an already established relationship with the researcher. On the other hand, a co-facilitator could make valuable observations during the interview and record them as field notes.

The development, sequencing and wording considerations of interview questions are like those related to questionnaires and should be reviewed prior to conducting the interviews. Interview schedules should also be pre-tested and assessed for reliability and validity. The pre-test is also valuable in terms of the readiness and skills of the interviewer.

Data obtained in structured interviews are usually recorded on the interview schedule or a separate coding sheet. The process of recording responses should be clear to the interviewer. Data obtained from semi-structured and unstructured interviews can be recorded on audio equipment, online recordings on Zoom or other software programs or video recordings. Field notes and logs are preferred record-keeping devices for interviews.

Training should be provided for all interviewers and should be carried out in groups so that each interviewer receives the same instructions. The more unstructured the interview, the greater the need for training and experience.

All interviews should occur at a time that is convenient for both researcher and interviewee. Adequate time is crucial to the completion of the interview schedules. Interviews may occur in a variety of settings – for example, a ward, clinic or school.

Regardless of the setting, the interviewer should seek as much privacy as possible for the interview. The time of the interview may never interfere with core business such as rendering patient care, teaching time or patients' rights. For example, a patient must not be taken out of the queue in the waiting room of a clinic, resulting in losing his or her place or the opportunity to receive treatment.

The interviewer can have a great deal of influence on the outcome of face-to-face interviews. Studies show that gender, ethnicity, accents and clothing influence answers provided by interviewees. In online or telephonic interviews, the interviewer's verbal mannerisms, such as tone of voice and dialect, can be a positive or negative factor in obtaining the interviewees' co-operation. Furthermore, an interviewer must always be cautioned against the possibility of showing a sense of superiority over the participant.

Scales

These self-report data-collection instruments ask respondents to record their attitudes or feelings on a continuum. A scale is composed of a set of numbers, letters or symbols that have rules and which can be used to 'locate' individuals on a continuum. There are different types of scales, the most common being semantic, differential, rating, summated rating, Likert, Guttman and visual analogue.

A Likert scale is an example of a summated rating scale which is frequently used to test attitudes or feelings. It is summative in that item scores are added to obtain the result. It consists of several declarative statements about the topic, with five or seven responses for each statement, ranging from 'strongly agree' to 'strongly disagree'. Items or questions can also be reversed, in other words asked twice in two different ways (positive and negative) to ensure a high score of consistency.

Figure 11.2 provides an example of one item/question in a Likert scale.

Statement 1	Healthcare professionals should practise therapeutic touch in patient care situations				
	Strongly disagree	Disagree	Uncertain	Agree	Strongly agree
	1	2	3	4	5

Figure 11.2 Example of a Likert scale

An approximately equal number of positively and negatively worded items should be included in a Likert instrument. To score it, the responses of all items are added to obtain a total score. The values obtained are treated as interval data. If five responses are used (as in Figure 11.2), scores on each item generally range from 1 to 5. If 20 items are included, the total score could vary between 20 and 100. A score of 1 is usually given to 'strongly disagree', and a score of 5 to 'strongly agree'. Negatively worded items are often reverse scored, in which case 'strongly disagree' is given a score of 5, and 'strongly agree' a score of 1.

Physiological measures

Because of the connections between physiological measures and clinical health sciences practice, many researchers use these measures. Among the most familiar are blood pressure values, blood values, urine values and electrocardiograms. Two of the greatest advantages of physiological measures are their precision and accuracy.

Other techniques

Vignettes

Vignettes are short, descriptive sketches of a situation or event to which participants must respond (Polit & Beck, 2022). Vignettes are also described as a variant of the case study method. Vignettes use short, systematically varied descriptions of situations or persons (called vignettes) to elicit the beliefs, attitudes or behaviours of respondents with respect to the presented scenarios. Synonyms for vignettes are anecdotes, illustrations, scenarios, sketches, narratives, pictures or stories.

A classic example is that of Ganong, Coleman and Riley (1988), who present hypothetical information about a pregnant woman to two groups of health sciences students in two sessions per group: one is a verbal description and the other a video of a healthcare professional interviewing the woman. The information is identical, except that the woman is married in the Group 1 version and unmarried in the Group 2 version. After hearing the verbal report, each group completes two scales. After seeing the video they complete another instrument. The married woman is rated more favourably than the unmarried woman on all subscales except activity. Furthermore, the students predicted that the unmarried woman would have a more difficult time if hospitalised than the married one. The use of vignettes enabled the researcher to distinguish the healthcare professionals' attitudes about married and unmarried women indirectly. Such an approach is more likely to reveal true attitudes than is a direct question, which often receives an answer that respondents think is socially acceptable.

Records and available data

A researcher need not collect new data to undertake a scientific investigation. Hospital records, admission charts, incident reports, care plan statements, students' test and examination results and sick leave records all constitute rich data sources. Access to records follows proper procedures that meet the ethical requirements of research. Informed consent and permission are based on the specific type of records, purpose of the study, and institutional and legal requirements.

Records serve as an economical source of information. They permit an examination of trends over time and eliminate the need for researchers to seek co-operation from participants. However, the use of records may be exposed to many sources of error.

The records may contain institutional biases, facts may be distorted, some facts may be omitted, record-keeping may be erratic, the collection of data may have been stopped for political or financial reasons, and some data are not readily available owing to their confidential nature.

Critical incidents

As with all data collection, the collection of critical incidents requires careful preparation, planning and practice. The critical incident technique is used in a variety of ways in health sciences research. It is a set of procedures for collecting direct observations of human behaviour in a way that facilitates potential usefulness in solving practical problems. An incident relates to any observable human activity sufficiently complete in itself to permit inferences to be made. For example, healthcare professionals can be asked to report incidents they observe which are effective or ineffective in meeting certain goals. A researcher may be interested in establishing factors that relate to giving a good patient report. Healthcare professionals could be asked to describe activities that result in an effective report being given by the nurse in charge of a ward. Analysis of the responses enables the researcher to compile a description of effective and ineffective report-giving. In another example, new mothers could be asked to identify the most stressful event that occurred during labour or delivery. The analysis of the experiences of the mothers enables the researcher to propose support strategies and best practices during labour.

Secondary analysis

Secondary analysis refers to studies where existing data from a previous or ongoing study is used to answer new questions or test new hypotheses that were not initially envisaged. This type of analysis is done in both qualitative and quantitative research. Grove, Gray and Burns (2018: 488) describe secondary analysis as any 'reanalysis' of data collected by another researcher or research team, or information collected by an organisation. Outcomes researchers use secondary data such as hospital discharge data to determine outcomes or patterns over a period of time or within a specific area.

Summary

In this chapter we focused on data-collection techniques. We discussed the five important questions that a researcher must pose when planning data collection and explored the most commonly used and some of the less frequently used techniques and methods. We provided the advantages and disadvantages of each technique; with this knowledge, the researcher should be able to select the most appropriate method for the study at hand.

Exercises

Complete these exercises:

1. You are interested in studying the experiences of adolescents who attend a primary healthcare clinic for family planning services. Argue the appropriateness of a structured versus an unstructured data collection technique.

2. An investigation of unemployed healthcare professionals is to be accomplished by means of an online questionnaire. Draft a covering letter to accompany the questionnaire.

3. A researcher is planning to study temper tantrums displayed by hospitalised children. Would you recommend they use a time sampling or an event sampling approach? Justify your choice.

4. What are the steps in instrument development? Explain how error can be reduced in this process.

5. What factors should the researcher consider when choosing a self-report method?

6. Identify the flaws in the following questions and suggest improvements:

   (a) How do you feel about surgery and holistic medicine?

   (b) Do you believe that being overweight is only due to overeating?

   (c) Do you often forget to take your prescribed medicine?

   (d) Do you support the statement made by the clinic nurse that patients 'do not adhere to treatment'?

7. Discuss the advantages, disadvantages and ethical implications of web-based questionnaires. Suggest suitable types of studies for this data-collection method.

8. Give an example of a study where vignettes could be used to collect data.

Data quality

This chapter covers factors that can affect reliability and validity in data collection. All researchers want to produce quality research. They want results to be meaningful, to reflect reality as accurately as possible, and to be replicable. Unfortunately, all measurement is accompanied by the possibility of error. No data-collection technique is perfect. It is therefore essential that researchers control for error and reduce error as much as possible.

Types of error

Two types of error can occur in the measurement process: random errors and systematic, or continuous, errors.

Random errors

A random (chance) error occurs due to arbitrary disturbances in performance on the measure. It is an unpredictable error which is unsystematic in nature and results in inconsistent data. These disturbances mean that an individual's score on the measure would be higher than their true score on one occasion, but lower than their true score on another. Random error can disturb the relationship between variables and make them weaker (Polit & Beck, 2022). Random errors thus directly affect data reliability. These errors can be caused by factors relating to the participant, the researcher, the environment or the instrument. For example, if a patient awaiting a root canal treatment at the dental clinic is requested to complete a questionnaire, the responses they give about their current stress levels are likely to differ from those they may have given under less stressful circumstances.

The difference between random error (sometimes referred to as random measurement error) and systematic error lies in the direction of the error. In random error the difference between the measured error and the true value error does not have a particular pattern or direction, and is therefore 'random' (Grove, Gray & Burns, 2018).

Systematic errors

A systematic (or continuous) error consistently affects the variable's measurement in the same way each time the measurement is done. This non-random bias impacts the reliability of a measure. It provides an incorrect measure of the variable, and the error will be the same for every participant. There are four types of systematic error, namely theoretical error, observational error, environmental error and instrumental error. Systematic error can be identified by comparing the results from your analysis to the standard. Standard data or known theoretical results serve as a reference to detect or determine the systematic error in the data. According to LoBiondo-Wood and Haber (2014), a systematic error always occurs in one direction. An example is a weight scale that consistently weighs a person 1 kg less than their actual body mass. The measurement appears to be reliable (as repeated measures will result in the same mass), but it is not valid.

Other examples are social desirability (where participants answer questions in a way that they perceive to be socially desirable, regardless of whether the answers are true), and acquiescent response sets (where participants consistently agree or disagree with the questions). These habits are always present in some people, and their responses will bias any questionnaire or interview (Terre Blanche, Durrheim & Painter, 2012). The researcher must therefore take special precautions to design their instrument to limit such errors.

Sources of measurement error

There are many sources of measurement error, and the most common are those caused by the participants, the researcher, the environment and the instrumentation.

Participant factors

A participant who is tired, sick, hungry, angry, irritable or confused may cause error in the instrumentation. In fact, any changing physical, emotional or psychological state can introduce error. The participants' awareness of the researcher's presence during observation changes behaviour because they know they are being studied (the Hawthorne effect); anonymity of responses in a self-report study and familiarity with the researcher may also cause bias. Power differentials between the researcher and participants are further causes of bias and error. Participants sometimes try to present themselves in the best way and manipulate their responses to this end. Recalling past events, experiences and behaviour selectively also influences the measurement of variables. The careful researcher ensures that the factors which could influence participants and their responses are controlled.

Researcher factors

The researcher can influence the results of the study in several ways. For example, their physical appearance, their clothing, their demeanour and their personal attributes could all play a role. In situations where the researcher or data collector is uninterested in the task, fatigued, impatient, bored, ill, subjective towards the participant for whatever reason or distracted may also contribute to random error. The researcher must thus attempt to put aside emotions during the data-collection process. In the case of the researcher's erroneous logic affecting the conceptualisation of a study, the results could be biased. The researcher could also record observations differently owing to perceptual differences and observer variations.

Environmental factors

Factors causing random error in measurement can stem from the physical environment in which the research occurs: weather, temperature, lighting, noise and interruptions all play a role in this. The researcher should ensure that the environment is conducive to testing and that all testing times and sites are similar.

Instrumentation factors

Some factors which cause random error derive from the instrument. For example, unclear questions or directions, inadequate sampling, question format, the order in which questions are asked and the way questions are worded can all be sources of random error. If a respondent does not know how to respond, they may choose to guess rather than give a true answer. The researcher should conduct a pre-test of the instrument, or a small-scale or pilot study, to find out if other sources are apparent.

Validity of data-collection instruments

Chapters 8 and 9 discussed internal and external validity. This chapter deals with the related topic of instrument validity. Instrument validity seeks to ascertain whether an instrument provides accurate measures given the context in which it is applied. Unless the researcher is certain that the instruments actually measure the things they are supposed to, they cannot be certain of what the results mean. For example, if they design a study to examine parenting skills, but use an instrument which measures general coping skills, the study's results are invalid. Similarly, if the researcher examines the relationship between effective healthcare and a particular kind of education, but uses an instrument which measures attitudes toward health sciences as a profession, the results could be misleading.

Content validity

Content validity is an assessment of how well an instrument represents all components of the variable to be measured, and always precedes data collection. When one or more component is neglected, the researcher cannot claim to be measuring whatever they are interested in. For example, if the researcher designs a questionnaire on individuals' responsibility to ensure their own health insurance, but forgets to ask about the financial status of the participant, the instrument is incomplete and therefore has poor content validity.

This type of validity is usually used when developing questionnaires, interview schedules or interview guides. The researcher constructing the instrument often bases their claim on a literature review. The literature review reveals the essential aspects of the variable which must be included in the content. Concepts should be clearly defined, and logical discussions thereof are required to prevent confusing or vague statements. The instrument is then presented to a group of experts for evaluation of its content validity. The evaluation assesses each item on the instrument about the degree to which the variable to be tested is represented, as well as the instrument's overall suitability for the specified purpose or use. In examining the variable the group assesses not only that which the instrument measures, but also that which it does not. Thus, the issue of how representative the questions are on the test of the phenomenon is foregrounded. Experts do not perform statistical measurements in judging content validity: the instrument is instead given to persons similar to respondents of that study to pre-test in terms of clarity and whether it measures the essential aspects of the relevant variables.

Face validity

Face validity is the least effective kind of instrument validity. The instrument appears to measure what it is supposed to and is essentially based on an intuitive judgement made by experts. The researcher may find the procedure useful in the instrument development process with regard to determining readability and clarity of content. For example, if participants indicate that the instrument is not relevant to their situation based on looking at it, then face validity is a problem. However, it should not be considered a satisfactory alternative to other types of validity.

Establishing face and content validity is just the first task in establishing the accuracy of the data-collection instrument. Before using the instrument in a new study the researcher should seek more objective means of establishing its validity.

Criterion-related validity

Criterion-related validity is a pragmatic approach to establishing a relationship between the scores on the instrument and other external criteria. The researcher can test whether an instrument measures what it is expected to by comparing it to another measure known to be valid. The other measure is known as the 'criterion measure'. Criterion-related validity is therefore when the scores obtained with a particular instrument are a good reflection of a 'gold standard' (an ideal measure of the construct measured) (Polit & Beck, 2022). If data collected using the instrument closely match data collected using the criterion measure, the researcher may conclude that the new instrument is also valid. The two data sets must be collected from the same participants. A new instrument often needs to be developed even if a valid one already exists because the existing valid instrument neither meets the research aims nor suits its design.

There are two kinds of criterion-related validity: predictive validity and concurrent validity.

Predictive validity

Predictive validity deals with future outcomes. It involves comparing the instrument results obtained from a particular population to an event, or a measure (criterion), which is expected to occur in that population in the future. For example, if a researcher finds evidence in the literature of a relationship between high stress and the onset of illness, they design an instrument to measure stress in adults 65 years or older and administer it to a large group of study participants. They predict which of the participants are more likely to develop illnesses in the coming year based on the results. At the end of the year the researcher can determine the accuracy of their prediction by correlating the scores obtained from the stress scale with the onset of illness for the total year in the participants.

Another example is provided by Bless, Higson-Smith and Sithole (2013). A researcher has evidence that students' motivation is directly related to their final marks. They develop a questionnaire to measure motivation and administer it to a large group of students. The researcher is able to predict which students will do well and which poorly in their final examinations. When the students write their final examination at year-end, the researcher can determine the accuracy of their predictions based on students' motivation at the start of the year.

A statistical test establishes the degree of correlation between the research instrument result and the criterion measure. However, the criterion measure may have resulted from variables other than those under investigation. In the example provided above, study variables such as different textbooks, study habits and other circumstances may have influenced the results. Predictive validity should thus only be used if the researcher is convinced that the variable under investigation has a clear criterion measure against which another instrument can be tested.

Concurrent validity

Concurrent validity differs from predictive validity in that the results of the new data-collection instrument are compared to those of a criterion measure at the same point in time. For example, a self-report measure of pain – the new instrument – may be compared with physiological measures of pain, such as pulse rate. Similarly, the results of a newly constructed behavioural checklist to measure healthcare professionals' job satisfaction could be compared with those of an established (and valid) job satisfaction instrument. A correlation between the results of the two tests would indicate concurrent validity for the checklist. The main difficulty with criterion-related validity in practice is finding a relevant criterion that is valid and reliable. Once the researcher has established a criterion, validity can be measured by correlating the test and criterion scores.

Construct validity

Construct validity measures the relationship between the instrument and the related theory. One could ask the question: 'What construct is the instrument actually measuring?' It is the most important and frequently used form of validity discussed thus far. Construct validity is useful mainly for measures of traits or feelings. It is more complex than criterion-related validity and is usually established over a period by several people, instead of by the instrument's originator alone. It is used to explore the relationship between the instrument's results and measures of the underlying theoretical concept(s).

Validity from divergence

Some researchers wish to measure a concept's opposite. An example could be a researcher who wishes to measure positive attitudes towards an event, for example, the hosting of a sport world cup, also measuring the negative attitudes towards it. By determining both ends of the attitude scale, the evidence of validity from divergence provides correlational information. If the divergent measure is negatively correlated with the other instrument, validity for each of the instruments is strengthened (Grove, Gray & Burns, 2018).

Validity from convergence

Grove, Gray and Burns (2018) also refer to evidence of validity from convergence. This is when a relatively new instrument is compared with an existing instrument, or with more than one instrument. Both instruments are administered and the results are correlated. If there is correlation between the two sets of measurement, the instruments are strengthened.

We will now consider some of the most common approaches used to determine construct validity (Grove, Gray & Burns, 2018; Polit & Beck, 2021).

Contrasted groups

Also referred to as the 'known-groups approach', this approach is carried out by comparing two groups. For example, a group of severely depressed people would be expected to have high scores on a depression checklist, whereas a group of those not suffering from depression would have low scores on the same checklist. The checklist (the data-collection instrument) can be given to both groups and the scores compared. If the instrument is valid, the mean score of these groups will be significantly different.

The multi-trait, multi-method approach

This approach is the preferred method of establishing construct validity. It is based on the two-fold premise that different measures of the same constructs should produce similar results, and that measures of different constructs should produce differing ones. To perform this type of test, the researcher must have access to more than one method of measuring the construct under study. Anxiety, for example, could be measured by:

- observing the participant's behaviour
- asking the participant about their anxious feelings
- recording blood-pressure readings
- administering an anxiety inventory.

The results of one of these measures should then be correlated with the results of each of the others in a multi-trait, multi-method matrix.

A variety of data-collection methods (such as self-report observation and collection of physiological data) can be used to test construct validity. A second requirement of the multi-trait, multi-method approach is that the researcher measures constructs from which they wish to differentiate the key construct, using the same measuring methods. For example, the researcher wants to distinguish anxious persons from calm ones. Since the two concepts are related, the researcher would therefore expect, on average, that persons who exhibited a high degree of anxiety would score poorly in terms of calmness. The point of including both concepts in a single validation study is to gather evidence that they are, in fact, distinct, rather than being two different labels for the same trait or characteristic.

Validity of qualitative data

Qualitative research methods do not lend themselves to statistical calculations of validity. However, this does not imply that qualitative researchers are not concerned with the quality of their data-collection techniques. The central question that determines the concept of validity and reliability addresses the issue of whether the measures used by the researcher yield data that reflect the truth. A number of authors focusing on qualitative research methods suggest data collection strategies that the researcher can employ to enhance the truthfulness or validity of qualitative results. Several such strategies were discussed in Chapter 9 and will be discussed in more detail under the section on trustworthiness later in this chapter.

Reliability of data-collection instruments

The reliability of the research instrument is another major concern for the researcher when they collect data. 'Reliability' refers to the degree to which an instrument can be depended upon to yield consistent results if used repeatedly over time on the same person, or if used by two researchers. The reliability of an instrument is indicated by a correlation measure that varies between 0 and 1. The nearer the measure is to 1, the higher the correlation. The three characteristics of reliability which are commonly evaluated are discussed below.

Stability

'Stability' of a research instrument refers to its consistency over time. It is measured by giving the same individuals an instrument on two occasions (within a relatively short period of time) and examining their responses for similarities. This method is termed 'test-retest reliability'. Problems with this technique include the fact that some persons may respond to the instrument the second time based on their memory of their first exposure to it. They may also undergo changes, particularly if the period of intervention is longer.

The test-retest technique is usually used in interviews and questionnaires. When observations are used, the test is called 'repeated observation'.

Internal consistency

Sometimes referred to as 'homogeneity', internal consistency addresses the extent to which all items on an instrument measure the same variable. This type of reliability is appropriate only when the instrument examines one concept or construct at a time. For example, if it is designed to measure emotional intelligence, all items on the instrument must consistently measure emotional intelligence. Other concepts frequently measured in health sciences are assertiveness, job satisfaction, burn-out, depression, self-esteem and autonomy.

The most common method employed to estimate internal consistency is the 'split-half' method. This is done by splitting the items on the instrument into two halves, and computing correlations between their scores. The halves can be divided by obtaining the scores on the first half of the test and comparing them with the scores on the second half, or by comparing odd-numbered items to even-numbered ones. Because the reliability of a measure is associated with the number of items, the split-half procedure tends to decrease the correlation coefficient.

Special statistical tests have been developed to provide measures of internal consistency for questionnaires. Cronbach's alpha coefficient is the test most frequently used to establish internal consistency. While it is useful for establishing reliability in a highly structured quantitative data-collection instrument, it is less effective in open-ended questionnaires or interviews, unstructured observations, projective tests, available data, or other qualitative data-collection methods and instruments.

Equivalence reliability

Tests of equivalence attempt to determine whether similar tests given at the same time yield the same results, or whether the same results can be obtained by using different observers at the same time. The former case is sometimes referred to as the use of 'parallel forms'. This requires the availability of alternative versions of a test or questionnaire examining the same concept. The researcher then administers the two instruments consecutively to the same participants and compares the results of the two tests statistically to determine the degree of association (or correlation) between them. This method is more commonly used in educational testing than in health sciences research.

However, it may be a useful approach in establishing the reliability of results obtained from knowledge-testing procedures when client-teaching methods are being investigated.

The latter case is frequently referred to as 'inter-rater reliability'. It is the method of testing for equivalence when the design calls for observations. Establishing inter-rater reliability is essential if more than one individual will be collecting data. The comparison of data obtained will provide evidence of the similarities (or dissimilarities) in the measurements or observations made by the various raters or observers. A reliable instrument should produce the same results if both observers use it in the same way. If the observations or measurements obtained on the same participants are statistically different between raters, there is a problem in ensuring inter-rater reliability.

Relationship between reliability and validity

Reliability and validity are closely related. The researcher needs to consider both when selecting a research instrument. There is no point in using an instrument that is not valid, however reliable it may be. Equally, if an instrument measures a phenomenon of importance, but the measurements are not consistent, it is of no use. In essence, reliability is a part of validity in that an instrument which does not yield reliable results cannot be considered valid. It is possible that an instrument can be used to collect reliable data, but the reliability of the method does not guarantee that the data collected are valid measures of research concepts. A valid measure is also an accurate and consistent, or reliable, one. Denscombe (2010: 268) points out that if the data are to be regarded as valid, the researcher must know that:

- The research instrument does not vary in the results it produces on different occasions when it is used.
- Respondents generally answer in a consistent way and provide the same kind of answers to similar questions.
- Different researchers would draw similar conclusions when analysing the same data.
- The findings will apply to other contexts and people.
- The analysis works or is correct in that the researcher can validate that the data analysis that was used is better than an alternative.

An important skill in developing (or finding) good measurement techniques involves being able to recognise a technique that is adequate in terms of both validity and reliability.

Trustworthiness

Chapter 9 discussed trustworthiness in terms of validity and reliability. 'Qualitative validity' refers to the employment of procedures to ensure accuracy of findings. The use of multiple strategies results in authenticity and credibility. Strategies recommended by Cresswell (2014) to ensure validity include:

- triangulating
- member checking to determine the accuracy of findings by referring the report on the analysed data back to the participants

- making detailed descriptions of data
- the researcher self-reflecting to clarify possible biases
- discussing contrary data as part of the identified themes
- engaging lengthily in the research setting to gain an in-depth understanding of the phenomenon under investigation
- peer debriefing
- external auditing.

'Qualitative reliability' refers to consistency across studies and researchers. This can be assured by documenting data accurately and comprehensively, checking transcripts for correctness, coders collaborating with co-coders through regular communication, and cross-checking codes and reaching inter-coder agreement (Cresswell, 2014).

Bearing this in mind, trustworthiness is now examined as a way of ensuring data quality (or rigour) in qualitative research, based on the model of Lincoln and Guba (1985). This model proposes four criteria for developing trustworthiness of a qualitative study: credibility, dependability, confirmability and transferability (Polit & Beck, 2021). Guba and Lincoln (1994) then added a fifth criterion, namely authenticity. Each of them is based on epistemological standards.

'Credibility' alludes to confidence in the truth of the data and the interpretation thereof. The investigation must be done so that the findings demonstrate credibility. Confidence in the truth can be established through the following techniques:

- **Prolonged engagement** by staying in the field until data saturation has been reached. In this way, the researcher gains an in-depth understanding of the phenomenon as well as specific aspects of the participants (such as perceptions or views, culture and experiences). It builds trust and rapport between researcher and participants.
- **Persistent observation** by consistently pursuing interpretations in various ways. This strategy is used during data collection. The researcher looks for multiple influences through a process of continual and tentative analysis and determines what counts and what does not.
- **Triangulation** by asking different questions, seeking different sources and using different methods. This includes collecting data about different events and relationships from differing points of view. Investigator triangulation is sometimes used during data coding or analysis.
- **Peer debriefing** by seeking the opinions of peers outside the study who have similar status or are colleagues (not novices or juniors) and who are experts in either the method or the phenomenon being studied. These colleagues should have a general understanding of the study and should be able to debate each step of the research process with the researcher.
- **Member checks** by assessing the intentionality of the participants, to correct obvious errors and to provide additional information. The emerging findings of the study are taken back to the participants for the interpretations of the data, as well as the adequacy thereof, to be discussed and confirmed.

- **Negative case analysis** by continually revising and refining a theory. This is done by including cases which appear to disconfirm the theory and continues until all cases are accounted for. Negative case analysis is a methodological approach in qualitative research, where the researcher searches for and discusses data that contradict the explanations emerging from the research.
- **Referral adequacy** by determining all materials available to document findings.

'Dependability' refers to the provision of evidence such that if it were to be repeated with the same (or similar) participants in the same (or similar) context, its findings would be similar. The term thus refers to the data's stability over time. This is the alternative to reliability as described in quantitative research. When dependability is absent, credibility cannot be attained. All techniques applied to ensure credibility also directly impact on dependability. Further techniques to ensure dependability are **stepwise replications**, in which all steps are replicated by two or more teams, who deal with the data independently and then compare the findings. In **inquiry audits**, the auditor examines documentations of critical incidents and the process of the investigation. Determining the acceptability of the investigation attests to its dependability. Thus, the data, findings, interpretations and recommendations are also examined to attest that the investigation is supported by data and is internally coherent, thereby establishing confirmability.

'Confirmability' refers to the potential for congruency of data in accuracy, relevance or meaning. It is concerned with establishing whether data represent the information provided by the participants, and that the interpretations are not fuelled by the researcher's imagination. The data must reflect the voice of the participants, and not the researcher's biases or perceptions. Techniques to enhance confirmability are inquiry audit, reflexivity and triangulation. **Reflexivity** refers to having an awareness that the researcher as an individual brings along to the inquiry, a unique set of values and beliefs, their own background and a professional identity. A strategy to maintain reflexivity in research is to keep a journal or diary. Thoughts and experiences during the inquiry are documented on a continuous basis. The researcher also records how previous experiences and readings are affecting the inquiry. In doing so, the researcher is able to probe deeper during data collection and gain a better understanding of the lifeworld of the participants.

'Transferability' refers to the ability to apply the findings in other contexts, or to other participants. The qualitative researcher is not primarily concerned with (statistically) generalising the findings, but rather with defining observations within the contexts in which they occur. Within qualitative research, demonstrating transferability of findings lies with those who wish to apply it in another context. Strategies to enhance transferability are detailed descriptions, purposive sampling and data saturation. **Thick descriptions** entail the collection and provision of sufficient detailed descriptions of data within a given context, and their reportage. The reader then makes a judgement about transferability. **Purposive sampling** maximises the range of specific information obtained from (and about) the particular context, by purposefully selecting participants in terms of knowledge of the phenomenon under investigation as well as the locations. Data saturation occurs when additional participants provide no new information, and when themes that emerge become repetitive. The sample is then considered adequate, and the data rich and thick.

'Authenticity' refers to the extent to which the researchers indicate a range of realities in a fair and true manner. A report must convey the experiences and emotions of the participants as they occur. The reader should develop an increased sensitivity to the issues being discussed and should be able to understand the lives being portrayed in the report with some sense of the participants' experiences and emotions.

Data enhancement strategies organised by phase of the study

To increase the confidence in the integrity of the findings of a study, Polit and Beck (2022) mention the following data enhancement strategies. These strategies are organised by phase of the study.

- During data collection the researcher engages in:
  - prolonged engagement and persistent observation
  - reflexive strategies
  - data and method triangulation
  - comprehensive recording of information
  - member checking.
- During coding and analysis the researcher engages in:
  - investigator triangulation
  - searching for disconfirming evidence and competing explanations
  - peer review and debriefing
  - inquiry audits.
- Strategies related to presentation:
  - thick and contextual description
  - researcher credibility.

Although not exhaustive, the strategies mentioned here should guide the researcher to carefully assess the steps taken to enhance the quality of the data.

Other factors affecting data quality

In addition to reliability and validity, the researcher must examine a number of other criteria before using a data-collection instrument.

Sensitivity

The 'sensitivity' of an instrument refers to its ability to discriminate. A sensitive instrument can detect change. Therefore, when evaluating data-collection instruments, the evaluator should consider whether the instrument is sensitive enough to ensure valid data are collected.

Efficiency

An 'efficient' instrument is one which requires minimum effort and expense but manages to measure with validity and reliability. A questionnaire or interview schedule should only be as long and as complex as necessary to achieve credible reliability and validity. A perfect instrument which is too complex and expensive to use will not collect much data. Both the researcher's and research participants' time should be considered. The costs of various techniques should be weighed. Only information deemed necessary for the research should be solicited. 'Nice to know' information must be omitted.

Appropriateness

'Appropriateness' refers to the extent to which research participants can meet the demands imposed by the instrument. The content of the instrument should be understood by the researcher and all participants. Furthermore, the instrument should be appropriate for the participants in terms of their ability and readiness to furnish the required data: age, literacy levels, health status, culture and language are all pertinent considerations. For example, English may not always be appropriate in a study where participants speak indigenous languages.

Ability to generalise

Generalisability refers to the researcher's expectations that instruments which are reliable and valid in one study will be found to be so in another. For example, an instrument tested for validity and reliability with undergraduate students would not necessarily be valid for use with hospitalised adolescents.

The pilot study and pre-test

To test the practical aspects of a study the researcher can conduct a pilot test or a pre-test. This is usually accomplished by including a few individuals who meet the inclusion criteria, but who will not form part of the sample. Data collected during this process are not included in the main study. In some cases, however, the researcher may include the data in the main study, provided no changes were necessary to the instrument and the participants in the pre-test meet all the inclusion criteria and were informed about it before the pre-test started (as part of their informed consent).

Sometimes referred to as a 'preliminary study', a pilot is a small-scale study conducted prior to the main study on a limited number of participants. It aims to investigate the feasibility of the proposed study and to detect possible flaws in its methodology. Design problems can also be identified. Inaccessibility to the sample is often detected, especially where a study is conducted in a rural, inaccessible area. By conducting a pilot study flaws that could have severe consequences for the study can be identified, whether of scientific value, rigour, time, money or effort.

Researchers sometimes decide not to conduct a pilot study, but test only certain aspects, such as the data-collection instrument. A pre-test is done to investigate for possible flaws in the instruments (such as ambiguous instructions or wording, inadequate time limits), as well as whether the variables defined by operational definitions are actually observable and measurable. This does not necessarily determine whether study participants understand what is required of them in terms of instructions, ambiguity of items and insensitivity or embarrassing items, however. Such a pre-test is especially useful if the researcher has compiled the measuring instrument specifically for the purpose of the research project. Discussing the outcomes is essential for understanding the identified flaws.

Pre-testing is not limited to quantitative research. A qualitative researcher (especially in instances where it is a novice researcher) may conduct a pre-test, not only to test the question(s) but also to determine their interviewing skills, logistical arrangements for an interview (such as the venue, recording and privacy) and the suitability of the data collection technique.

The time and effort expended in conducting a pilot study or in pre-testing the instrument is well spent, as pitfalls and errors that may prove costly in the actual study can be identified and avoided.

Measurement evaluation

It is essential that the measurement methods described in a study are evaluated. The thoroughness and appropriateness of the measurement assessment are critical to the study's results. If the measures used are flawed or if insufficient precautions have been taken to avoid errors, the findings are not likely to be meaningful.

A checklist for evaluating the measurement aspects of quantitative and qualitative studies is presented below.

☐ Are the conceptual and operational definitions of the variables appropriate and related?

Quantitative data

☐ Are the instruments for data collection clearly described, and are there any indications in the report of efforts the researcher made to minimise errors?

Qualitative data

☐ Are the efforts that the researcher made to enhance or evaluate the trustworthiness of the data discussed clearly, and in enough detail? If not, is there any other information that allows researchers to conclude the data are credible?

☐ How did the researcher assess the reliability of the data-collection methods? Is/are the method(s) used clearly described and appropriate, or should an alternative method have been used? Is the reliability adequate?

☐ Which precautions did the researcher use and which strategies did they employ to enhance or evaluate the data's trustworthiness? How adequate were the procedures? Could alternative procedures have been used more profitably?

☐ How was validity assessed? Was/ were the method(s) used appropriate, or should an alternative method have been used? Does the validity of the instrument appear to be adequate?

☐ Were the statistical procedures used to assess the reliability and validity of the study reported in enough detail?

☐ How much faith can be placed in the results of the study, based on the information provided by the researcher?

Summary

In this chapter we presented an overview of the factors that may affect the quality of data collected in a research study. Few, if any, measuring instruments are infallible – we explained how errors can occur in studies. We discussed several methods for assessing reliability and validity, and briefly described other factors affecting data quality. Having provided an overview of the pilot study as the method for testing the practical aspects of a study, including its feasibility, the chapter ended with a checklist that the researcher can use to evaluate the measurement aspects of a study.

Exercises

1. The following research descriptions refer to research which may yield unreliable data:
   'Patient satisfaction about hospital services on the day of their discharge.'
   'Perceptions of older persons living in care facilities on efficiency of home-based care givers.'
   'The use of an instrument developed for first-year healthcare students on hospitalised teenagers.'

   (a) From these descriptions, indicate factors which may be responsible for unreliability.

   (b) How could reliability be enhanced in each of the examples?

2. Identify some examples of concurrent validity and predictive validity related to health sciences research practice.

3. Search for a study reporting on a quantitative study. Assess whether validity and reliability were ensured and justify your answer.

4. Explain what the multi-trait, multi-method of construct validity measures.

5. Draw up a table to indicate the various criteria for trustworthiness and indicate how researchers can ensure that all criteria are met.

6. Search for an article reporting on a qualitative study. Critique the section describing the trustworthiness of the study.

Data analysis

This chapter focuses on what to do with collected data. Since it would be impractical for the researcher to individually list each piece, they must choose methods of exploring and organising raw data, as well as analysing and interpreting it, to give the data meaning (Gray, Grove & Sutherland, 2017). 'Analysis' refers to separating something into its component parts. By organising quantitative data in various ways, the researcher gets an idea of the patterns, outliers and missing data. Spreadsheets allow the researcher to sort data, to search for specific data, to recode and graph data, to perform basic calculations, and to ask 'What if?' (Leedy & Ormrod, 2010: 289). When exploring data in qualitative research, it is vital for the researcher to be immersed in them.

Several techniques are used to display data and they are all aimed at answering the research questions. This phase (or step) is usually referred to as 'data analysis' and requires careful planning. It entails categorising, ordering, manipulating and summarising the data, and describing them in meaningful terms.

There are various strategies for analysis. Studies commonly rely on either narrative or statistical strategies in conjunction with graphic or pictorial ones. The strategy type depends on the study design, types of variables, the method of sampling and the method by which the data are collected and measured. A descriptive or qualitative research design (or unstructured questions in other designs) often elicits qualitative data of considerable depth. The narrative strategy is the strategy of choice for analysing the data. Data collected by means of quantitative designs use statistical strategies, but may in addition use strategies which are also used in qualitative analysis.

These strategies are not mutually exclusive. In other words, by using one method, researchers do not exclude another. They can use methods simultaneously to make a stronger case when addressing the research question. The researcher's preference (which is based on their philosophical beliefs and experience) will often influence the choice of strategy. However, it is important for the researcher to remember that if the analysis strategy is not logically consistent with the type of inquiry (and with the level of the data), the answers will be flawed and the usefulness of the results doubtful. The researcher should also consider that data analysis must be planned before data are collected. Without a plan, data which are unsuitable, insufficient or excessive may be collected.

Analysis of quantitative data

Statistics is a powerful tool when analysing quantitative data. Moreover, quantitative data is classified according to the level of measurement, or measurement scale, into nominal, ordinal and interval categories. The ratio level is omitted because both interval and ratio data use the same types of statistical analysis (Chapter 11 refers).

Without the aid of statistics, quantitative data would be a chaotic mass of numbers. Statistical methods enable researchers to reduce, summarise, organise, manipulate, evaluate, interpret and communicate quantitative data.

Descriptive statistics are used to explain and summarise data, and thus indicate what the data set looks like. These statistics convert and condense a collection of data into an organised visual representation in a variety of ways so that the data have some meaning. A descriptive approach employs measures such as frequency distributions (how many?), measures of central tendency (what is the midpoint or average?), dispersion or variability (how is the data spread?), and measures of relationships (how do variables correlate?). An example would be the statistics of a group of people showing their demographics such as age, gender and home language.

Inferential statistics use sample data to make inferences about the study's population from a smaller sample, and thus have a different function to descriptive statistics. They also help the researcher to determine whether a difference found between two groups (such as an experimental group and a control group) is a genuine difference, or whether it is merely a 'chance difference' which occurs because a non-representative sample is chosen from the population. In an inferential approach 'P' values – that is, the probability that the outcome is due to chance – are used to communicate the significance (or non-significance) of the differences. Furthermore, inferential statistics facilitate the testing of hypotheses. Such statistics include the chi-square test, t-test, analysis of variance, analysis of co-variance, factor analysis and multi-variate analysis.

An example of inferential statistics would be where the incomes of female healthcare professionals and male healthcare professionals are investigated. Based on the results, one could infer that the one group earns more than the other group.

Choosing appropriate statistical procedures

Not all researchers in the healthcare professions have enough knowledge about statistics. The services of a statistician may therefore be of vital importance. When consulting a statistician, the researcher describes the study's purpose, the research question(s), the hypotheses, aims/purpose and objectives, the study design and the level of measurement. While some research students may have access to free statistical consultation and services, in cases where they do not, it is important to include the costs of statistical analysis in the study's budget. Important decisions that must be made relate to the nature of the data and what the researcher wants to know. Careful preparation is needed before a statistician is consulted. It is good practice to consult a statistician from the development phase of the instrument to the finalisation of the data analysis and reporting. The researcher must be prepared to answer the statistician's questions, which may include:

- What do you want to know?
- How do you want to treat outliers?
- Are the variables dichotomous, and how do you want them to be treated?
- Do you want to treat ordered categories of data as interval data?
- Can you assume that data you categorised in intervals is normally distributed in the population?
- How many dependent variables did you use?
- Do you want to analyse relationships between variables or between individual cases?

The two categories of statistical methods are discussed in greater detail below.

Descriptive statistics

Descriptive statistics explain and summarise data. They can be subdivided according to the summary functions they perform.

Frequency distributions (f)

'Frequency' refers to the number of times a result occurs. Frequencies are obtained by counting the occurrence of scores or values represented in the data. A frequency distribution is a systematic arrangement of the lowest to the highest scores, linked with the number of times the score occurs. Each score can be listed separately or the results grouped. This means that the results are subdivided into classes (or collections) of scores, which are grouped together. The extent of a class is determined by its boundaries.

For example, when classifying according to age, the classes may be 0–9, 10–19, 20–29, etc. The class 0–9 reflects the number of children up to 9 years of age, the class of 10–19 reflects the number of individuals whose ages range from 10 to 19, and so on. It is important that classes be mutually exclusive and do not overlap – thus the classes should not be 0–10, 10–20, 20–30, etc.

Frequency distributions are appropriate for interval and ratio data. Frequency counts are appropriate for nominal and ordinal data and are obtained by counting the occurrence of each observation in a category.

Examples of organising data according to level of measurement

Some examples of the organisation of data according to levels of measurement are discussed below.

Example 1: Nominal data

In the case of **nominal data**, a researcher is interested in investigating whether more men than women suffering from tuberculosis were admitted to Tembisa Hospital in 2022. The investigation involves counting the number of cases falling under each sex. If there were 50 patients, of whom 10 were male and 40 female, the data could be presented as shown in Table 13.1, which displays the following conventions in tabulating data:

- The table as a whole and the categories must be clearly and fully labelled, so that readers can unambiguously interpret what they are observing.
- The label 'frequency (f)' of cases or measurements falling into a given category.
- The 'n' represents the total number of cases or measurements in a sample.
- The label 'N' represents the number of cases in a population.

Table 13.1 Frequency count of tuberculosis patients' sex admitted to Tembisa hospital during 2022

Sex	Frequency (f)
Male (M)	10
Female (F)	40
	N = 50

Example 2: Ordinal data

Ordinal data are represented by counting the number of cases, or the frequency, of each ordered rank up a scale. A co-researcher is involved in evaluating the efficacy of a new analgesic versus traditional treatment. A post-test-only control group design is used. The experimental group receives the new analgesic, while the control group is given the traditional treatment. Twenty patients are randomly assigned to each group. Pain intensity is assessed by the patients' pain reports five hours after minor surgery, on the following scale:

```
5 – excruciating pain
4 – severe pain
3 – moderate pain
2 – mild pain
1 – no pain
```

The raw data are as follows:

> ▨ Experimental group: 3, 4, 5, 3, 3, 3, 4, 2, 1, 3, 2, 1, 3, 4, 5, 2, 3, 3, 3, 3
> ▨ Control group: 5, 4, 4, 4, 5, 3, 4, 3, 2, 4, 4, 2, 4, 5, 3, 4, 4, 4, 5, 5

Once the results are tallied, data can be presented in a frequency table (Table 13.2 refers). Thus, once the data have been tabulated the outcome of the investigation can be seen. In this example the pain reported by the experimental group is less than that of the control group. When tallying raw data, it is helpful to use the familiar 'gate method' of recording frequencies: four vertical lines are listed for the first four occurrences of a score, and a slash is used to indicate the fifth occurrence. This procedure is repeated until all scores are recorded.

Table 13.2 Reported pain intensity of patients following traditional and new analgesic treatments

Pain intensity	Experimental groups (analgesic) f	Control group (traditional) f
1	2	–
2	3	2
3	10	3
4	3	10
5	2	5
	n = 20	n = 20

Example 3: Interval or ratio data

In the case of **interval** or **ratio data**, an example of patients who are routinely weighed on admission to hospital is used. The researcher must summarise the individual mass of 50 patients who were admitted to a surgical ward over a specific period of time. Their individual mass (the raw data) are as follows (to nearest kilogram):

> 75, 67, 76, 71, 73, 86, 72, 77, 80, 75, 80, 96, 93
>
> 75, 73, 83, 81, 82, 73, 92, 81, 87, 76, 84
>
> 78, 79, 99, 100, 88, 77, 71, 76, 75, 83, 66, 79
>
> 95, 85, 77, 87, 90, 73, 72, 68, 84, 69, 78, 77, 84, 94

Once the results are tallied, they can be presented in a frequency table (see Table 13.3). It is easier to understand the data by studying the table than by looking at the raw data. Evidently, frequency distributions and frequency counts present useful data summaries as they provide a much clearer picture of the results.

Table 13.3 Grouped frequency distribution of patients' mass in each ward

Class interval f	f
96–100	3
91–95	4
86–90	5
81–85	9
76–80	13
71–75	12
66–70	4
	n = 50

Simple descriptive statistics

Once the data have been summarised in a frequency distribution, it is useful to make comparisons concerning relative frequencies of scores falling into specific categories. Simple descriptive statistics used for this purpose are ratios, proportions, percentages and rates.

Ratios are statistics which express the relative frequency of one set of frequencies, 'A', in relation to another, 'B'. The formula for ratio is:

$$\text{Ratio} = \frac{A}{B}$$

Therefore, the ratio of males to females for the data presented in Table 13.1 is:

$$\text{Ratio (males to females)} = \frac{10}{40} = 0.25$$

$$\text{Ratio (females to males)} = \frac{40}{10} = 4.0$$

A proportion is a part of a whole and is calculated by placing the frequency of one category over that of the total numbers in the sample or population. For example, if a pizza is cut into eight equal slices, each slice is a proportion and can be written as ⅛ or 0.125. In Table 13.1, the proportion of males is as follows:

$$\frac{10}{50\ (10 + 40)} = \frac{1}{5} \text{ or } 0.2$$

A percentage is the number of parts per 100 that a certain portion of the whole represents. Proportions can be transformed into percentages by multiplying by 100. In the case of Tembisa Hospital, the percentage of males admitted with tuberculosis would be:

$$0.2 \times 100 = 20\%$$

In the pain intensity example, the percentage of people experiencing excruciating pain in the experimental groups in Table 13.2 is:

$$\frac{2}{20} \times 100 = 20\%$$

The two rates commonly used in epidemiological studies are **incidence rates** and **prevalence rates**. When summarising the results of an epidemiological investigation, the researcher commonly compares the number of disease cases with the size of the population at risk. They do this by calculating rates.

The incidence rate of a disease over a period of time is:

$$\frac{\text{number of new cases over the period}}{\text{population at risk}}$$

For example, in the town of Stanger the number of new leukaemia cases in 2021 was 289. The total number of leukaemia cases on 30 June 2021 was 3 492. The population of Stanger at the time was 176 000. Thus, the incidence rate for leukemia per 100 000 is:

$$\frac{289}{176\,000} \times 100\,000 = 164.2$$

The prevalence rate of a disease at a particular point in time is:

$$\frac{\text{total number of cases of the disease at the time}}{\text{population at risk}}$$

The prevalence rate of leukaemia per 100 000 people from Stanger on 30 June 2021 is:

$$\frac{3\,492}{176\,000} \times 100\,000 = 1984.1$$

All five of these simple descriptive statistics were obtained by the mathematical manipulation of raw data.

Measures of central tendency

Measures of central tendency are statistics or numbers expressing the most typical or average scores in a distribution. The **mean, median** and **mode** are measures of central tendency.

The **mean** is the arithmetical average of all the scores in a distribution. To obtain the mean, the researcher adds all the scores together and divides the total by the total number of scores. For example, the researcher assesses pain levels and obtains the following six scores on the pain scale: 12, 17, 14, 5, 12, 3. The mean would be:

$$\frac{\text{(the sum of all the scores)}}{\text{(the total number of scores)}} = \frac{63}{6} \text{ or } 10.5$$

The mean is appropriate for interval and ratio data. It is considered the most stable measure of central tendency if the distribution is normal. If it is not, the mean will not present an accurate picture of the distribution.

The **median** is the midpoint score or value in a group of data ranked from lowest to highest. Half of the scores are above the median and half are below. If the number of scores or values is uneven, that is, odd, the median is the middle score or value. If the number of scores or values is even, the median is the midpoint between the two middle values and is found by averaging them. If the pain scores, which are used for calculating the mean, are ranked, the result is as follows:

$$3 \; 5 \; 12 \; 12 \; 14 \; 17$$

Thus, the median for these scores is:

$$\frac{12 + 12}{2} = 12$$

The median is the best value of central tendency for ordinal data. It is also appropriate for interval and ratio data. It presents a more accurate picture when the distribution is curved.

The **mode** is the value or score which occurs most frequently in a distribution. In the example of scores on the pain scale 12 is the score that occurs most frequently – hence the mode is 12. If a distribution has only one mode (as is also the case in this example), it is referred to as 'unimodal'. If there are two modes, the distribution is known as 'bimodal'. If there are more than two, it is referred to as 'multimodal'. The mode can be used with every level of measurement. Although it is not the best measure of central tendency, it is the most appropriate measure for nominal data.

Measures of variability

Measures of variability describe how widespread values or scores are in a distribution. Two distributions with identical means could differ in terms of how spread out the data are, for example, how different people are from one another. For example, using the example of pain mentioned above – the pain scales of patients in two different wards both have a mean score of 10.5. In the orthopaedic ward the scores could have a wider range of scores, with some above 17 and some below 3. In the surgical ward there are few low or high scores. The orthopaedic ward is more heterogeneous (more varied) than the surgical ward, and the surgical ward is more homogeneous than the orthopaedic ward. The index of variability is computed to show the extent to which scores in a distribution differ from one another, thus showing the index of variability.

While the mean, median and mode describe something about the middle of a number set, the variation among the numbers shows whether or not scores cluster around the middle (with few scores at either extreme). The three statistics commonly used to indicate the numerical value of variability are the **range**, the **variance** and the **standard deviation**.

The **range** is the simplest method for examining variation among scores and refers to the difference between the smallest and largest values in a distribution. Using the pain scores example, the total range would be 17 minus 3, or 14. The range is affected by extreme cases and gives no indication of what lies between the highest and lowest scores. The range can be used with ordinal, interval and ratio data. However, its usefulness is limited because one extreme score can drastically change the range.

The **variance** is defined as the sum of the squared deviations about the mean, divided by the total number of values. This measure of variability or dispersion is equal to the standard deviation and is an intermediate value used in calculating the standard deviation.

The **standard deviation** is the most widely used measure of variability when interval or ratio data are described. It indicates how values vary about the mean of the distribution and is defined as the square root of the variance. Two sets of results with the same mean may differ considerably in distribution, but the standard deviation quantifies this difference. The greater the standard deviation, the more spread scores are in relation to the mean in a distribution. Textbooks on statistics provide a variety of calculable formulae to derive them. Furthermore, the widespread use of computers and calculators makes a discussion of these formulae superfluous.

The **normal curve** or **normal distribution** is a special kind of curve that represents the theoretical distribution of population scores. With regard to the curve, 'normal' is a mathematical term used in the sense that a normal distribution of variables is frequently found in biological, behavioural and clinical sciences. Variables such as blood pressure, height and weight are normally distributed in the population. For example, while a few extremely short and a few extremely tall people do exist, most people are within a few centimetres of each other in height.

For a frequency curve to approximate the normal curve, a fairly large number of values is needed, that is, at least 30. The normal curve is bell-shaped and symmetrical, with maximum height at the mean. The mean, median and mode are equal. Most of the values cluster around the mean. A few values occur on both extremes of the distribution curve. An additional characteristic of the normal curve is that a fixed percentage of the scores falls within a given distance of the mean.

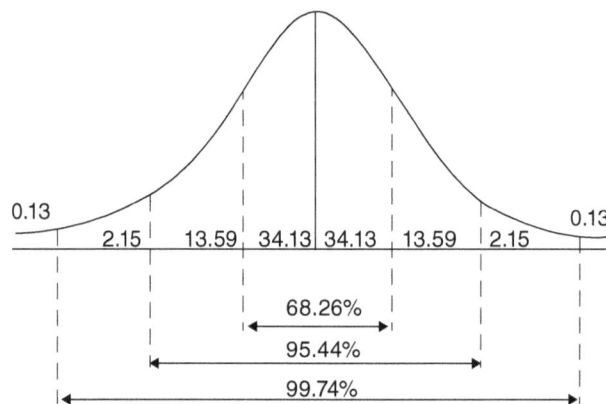

Figure 13.1 Percentage of the normal distribution between the mean and major points

As depicted in Figure 13.1, the following always holds true for a normal distribution:

- Approximately 68.26% of observations are located between the mean and one standard deviation on either side of it.
- Approximately 95.44% are located within two standard deviations of the mean on either side of it.
- Approximately 99.74% of observations are within approximately three standard deviations of the mean.
- This leaves 0.26% beyond three standard deviations, that is, 0.13 on either side.

What makes the normal distribution curve so useful is that in research on any normally distributed phenomenon the researcher can use the properties of the curve for making inferences and testing hypotheses. Once the mean and standard deviation of the data set are known, it is possible for them to determine precisely the proportion of observations between any two values.

In order to make comparisons between groups, standard scores rather than raw scores should be used. Once the mean and standard deviations for a given distribution have been calculated, any raw score can be transformed into a standard, or 'Z' score. The standard score represents by how many standard deviations a specific score is above or below the mean. A Z score of 1.5 means that it is 1.5 standard deviations above the mean, whereas a score of –2 means that the observation is 2 standard deviations below the mean. By utilising Z scores, the researcher can compare results from scales that utilise different units, such as height and mass.

Measures of relationship

Measures of relationship concern the correlation between variables. The concept of correlation is used when the researcher wants to determine the nature and extent of the relationship between variables: for example, a researcher wishes to establish the relationship between weight gain over a six-month period and the average daily calorie intake among a group of tuberculosis patients, or between the amount of time spent with a student in remedial teaching and the number of tests the student fails during that time. These data would be gathered on a group of patients or students. The researcher would need to know whether the two variables vary together, and would pose questions like: 'When tuberculosis patients increase their calorie intake, do they gain weight or not?' or, 'When time spent with students during remedial teaching increases, does the failure rate in tests increase or decrease?'

An important approach to drawing correlations is to examine the data and determine their nature and characteristics, and then select a correlational technique suitable for the data type (Gray, Grove & Sutherland, 2017; Leedy & Ormrod, 2010; Polit & Beck, 2021).

There are several ways to determine relationships such as these. We will now briefly explore correlation coefficients, scattergrams and contingency tables.

A correlation coefficient is a descriptive statistic or number that expresses the magnitude and direction of the association between two variables. To demonstrate that two variables correlate, the researcher must obtain measures on both for the same participants or events. For instance, the researcher obtains measures of tuberculosis patients' weight over a period of time (perhaps six months) along with their calorie intake over the same period.

Several types of correlation coefficients are used in statistics:

Table 13.4 Types of correlation coefficients used in statistics

φ (phi)	Both variables are measured on a nominal scale
ρ (rho) or Spearman's rank	Both variables are measured on, or transformed into, ordinal scales
r or Pearson's correlation coefficient	Both variables are measured on an interval or ratio scale

All of the correlation coefficients listed above are appropriate for quantifying linear relationships between variables. Regardless of which correlation coefficient the researcher employs, these statistics share the following characteristics:

- Correlation coefficients are calculated from pairs of measurements on variables X and Y for the same group of individuals.
- A positive correlation is denoted by + (a plus sign), and a negative correlation by – (a minus sign). A positive correlation means that the two variables tend to increase or decrease together. A negative correlation denotes an inverse relationship and indicates that as one variable increases, the other decreases.
- The values of the correlation coefficient range from +1 to –1, where +1 implies a perfect positive correlation, 0 implies no correlation and –1 implies a perfect negative correlation.

To obtain a visual representation of the relationship between two variables, the researcher plots the values obtained on a **scattergram**. A scattergram is a graphic presentation of the paired scores for each participant on the two variables. Pairs of scores are plotted on a graph by placing dots indicating where each pair of Xs and Ys intersects. If the pattern extends from the lower left corner to the upper right, a positive correlation is indicated. If the dots are distributed from the upper left corner downwards toward the lower right, a negative correlation exists. When the dots are scattered all over the graph, no relation exists between the two variables. The scattergrams in Figure 13.2 illustrate different correlations.

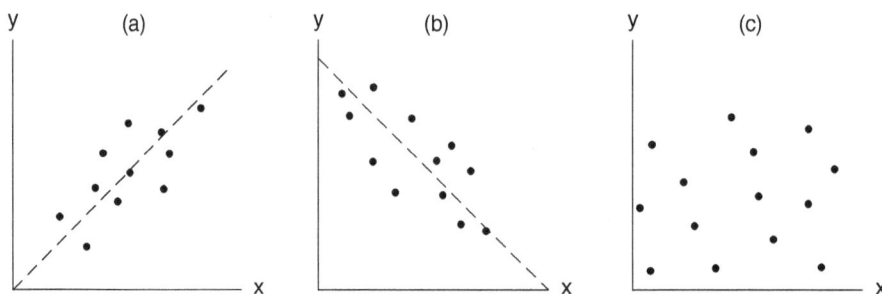

Figure 13.2 Scattergrams representing (a) a positive, (b) a negative, and (c) a case of no relationship between two variables

If data are nominal, relationships cannot be depicted on a scattergram. No actual scores are available in nominal data, but frequencies of the occurrence of the values are presented. A contingency table (also called a 'cross-tabulation table') is a means of visually displaying the relationship between sets of nominal data. For example, the researcher wishes to determine whether or not there is a relationship between gender and smoking. Table 13.5 depicts the data gathered on 50 male and 50 female participants.

Table 13.5 is called a 2 × 2 contingency table, because there are two variables, and each has two categories. If smoking had been divided into three categories, such as (a) 'never smoke', (b) 'smoke occasionally' and (c) 'smoke frequently', the table would have been called a 2 × 3 table.

Table 13.5 A 2 × 2 contingency table

Sex	Smoke regularly	Do not smoke regularly	Total
Male	30	20	50
Female	25	25	50
Total	55	45	100

The data in Table 13.5 seem to indicate that more men smoke than women. Further calculations must be done to determine whether or not the relationship between these variables is significant. The chi-square statistic is the statistic that would be calculated in this case.

If researchers want to describe and summarise the data they have obtained, they use descriptive statistics. If they want to infer, or draw conclusions about something, they use inferential statistics.

Reliability and validity affect correlation coefficients (Leedy & Ormrod, 2010: 275). If the researcher uses an instrument that has poor reliability and validity, the calculated correlation coefficients can be misleading and/or false.

Correlation does not show a cause–effect relationship. There might be a correlation between poverty and tuberculosis, but that does not mean that poverty causes tuberculosis. Obviously, if there is a strong correlation between two variables, the researcher may question whether one is caused by the other, but then they design a study to test the hypothesis. Only experimental studies can test a cause–effect relationship.

Inferential statistics

Inferential statistics enable a researcher to infer from a sample to a large population in order to estimate the population's parameters and test hypotheses (Leedy & Ormrod, 2010: 275). There are two kinds of inferential statistical tests: parametric and non-parametric.

Parametric statistics

Parametric statistics are applied to data where the following assumptions have been made:

● The variables of concern must be normally distributed within the targeted population.

- The selected sample must be representative of the target population and is thus a random sample.
- The variables are measured by an interval or ratio scale.
- The variances of groups compared should be approximately the same.
- The tests require estimates of parameters, for example, mean and standard deviation.

The most common parametric statistical tests used in health sciences research are the t-test and analysis of variance.

The **t-test** is used when the researcher wishes to compare the means of two groups in order to determine whether the differences between means are significant or caused by chance. There are two forms of t-test: one is used with independent samples, and the other with dependent samples. Samples are independent when there are two separate groups, such as an experimental group and a control group, and there is no association between their scores. Samples are dependent when the participants from the two groups are paired in some manner. For example, when the same participants are assessed on a given characteristic before and after an intervention, the sample is considered dependent. Dependent data are also obtained if each participant in one group is matched with a participant in another group on some variable, such as age or mass. The form of the t-test that is used with a dependent sample may be termed 'paired dependent', 'matched' or 'correlated'. Separate formulae are used to calculate the independent t-test and the dependent t-test.

Analysis of variance (ANOVA) is an extension of the t-test, which permits the researcher to compare more than two means simultaneously. ANOVA uses variances to calculate a value that reflects the differences between two or more means. When using ANOVA, the researcher calculates an F statistic or ratio. The larger the F value, the greater the variation or difference between the groups compared with the variation within the groups. If a statistically significant difference is found, other tests – called 'post-hoc comparisons', for example, Sheffe's or Tukey's tests – can be used to determine which of the means differ significantly. Regression statistics examine how effectively one or more variables allow the researcher to predict the value of others, such as the dependent variable. Factor analysis, on the other hand, examines the correlations between several variables and identifies clusters of highly interrelated variables that might reflect underlying factors within the data. Structured equation modelling (SEM) is used to examine the correlations between a number of variables in order to identify possible causal relationships (Leedy & Ormrod, 2010: 282). These tests do not fall within the scope of this textbook. Should your research require such analyses, please be guided by a statistician and make sure that you understand the meaning of each test.

Non-parametric statistics

Non-parametric statistics (also referred to as 'distribution-free' statistical tests) are applied to data where no assumptions are made regarding the normal distribution of the targeted population. These statistics are usually applied when variables have been measured on a nominal or ordinal scale. The chi-square is one of the most widely used non-parametric statistical tests in health sciences research. It is appropriate for comparing sets of data in the form of frequencies. Other examples of non-parametric tests are the Mann-Whitney test, which is an alternative to the independent form of the t-test, the Wilcoxon test for correlated samples, which is an alternative to the dependent form of the t-test, and the Kruskal-Wallis test, which is an alternative to ANOVA for comparing significant differences between several groups.

When using inferential statistical techniques to test a hypothesis, the researcher must be well acquainted with several statistical concepts, such as the probability or 'p' value or level of significance, degrees of freedom, critical values, one-tailed and two-tailed tests of significance, and type I and type II errors. You can consult statistical textbooks for clarification of these terms.

To choose the most appropriate inferential procedure for a study, the researcher must consider several factors:

- Am I testing for differences or for relationships?
- What is the level of measurement of the variables – nominal, ordinal, interval or ratio?
- Does the level of measurement permit the use of parametric statistics?
- What is the size of the sample?
- How was the sample selected?
- How many groups or sets of scores are being compared?
- Are the observations or scores dependent or independent?

In testing hypotheses the researcher plans the study carefully by using a large sample, valid and reliable measures, and parametric rather than non-parametric statistics. These strategies help the researcher to avoid errors in hypothesis testing.

Use of graphics

As Figure 13.1 illustrates, in addition to statistical tests, the use of graphic displays is recommended for almost every type of data. Graphics can effectively convey information related to data collected in a study and can be constructed in various ways. They appeal to the reader visually and invite them to analyse the data more closely than a written description. To be valuable, graphics must be accurate, simple and clear. They should represent the ideas and data presented in the research report well. Graphs should also fit the type of data collected – for example, bar charts and pie diagrams are generally used for nominal data, while histograms and frequency polygons are used for interval and ratio data. Information on the various types of graphs and how to plot them can be obtained in any statistical textbook.

Interpretation of quantitative data

A study's findings should be related to the original problem and research question. They can then be related to pre-existing literature, concepts, theories and research – creating a dialogue between findings and the literature. Furthermore, the researcher must determine whether the findings have practical significance. They might be statistically significant without being clinically significant and determining this helps the researcher in deciding whether to recommend changes in practice or not. Lastly, the researcher reflects on the limitations, as well as the strengths, of the study. No study is perfect.

Analysis of qualitative data

The data in qualitative research is non-numerical and is usually presented in the form of written material, video recordings, audio recordings, drawings and photographs. Analysis of data in qualitative studies therefore involves an examination of text rather than the numbers considered in quantitative studies. Frequently, a large amount of data in the form of text are gathered, which makes analysis time-consuming. Researchers using qualitative approaches tend to spend a lot of time reflecting on possible meanings and relationships of the data. This type of analysis is described as a 'hands-on' process during which the researcher becomes immersed in the data. It is also sometimes referred to as 'dwelling on' the data.

Generally, data analysis is not a separate distinct step in the qualitative research studies process, but it is done concurrently with data collection – unlike quantitative research analysis – which does not begin until all the data have been collected. The various forms of qualitative approaches have different forms of analysis. Nevertheless, many qualitative researchers use a series of common steps for analysing their data, which begins at the start of the data-collection phase. Breaking down qualitative data in steps helps the researcher to understand it better, but may create the impression that it is only done when all the data have been collected.

Data management involves converting the masses of data into smaller, more manageable segments. The data analysis process therefore starts with managing and organising the qualitative data. This first step allows the researcher to become immersed in the data. Data needs to be in a form that can be analysed: for example, interviews need to be transcribed and proofed against the recorded interview. In online data collection, the advantage is that interviews are recorded and transcribed at the same time. The transcribed version is therefore available immediately. The transcriptions can also be downloaded or copied directly into a computer-assisted qualitative data analysis software program (if used). During the analysis process, the researcher makes reflective and marginal remarks to understand what is happening. This phase is also referred to as data cleaning.

Field notes form part of the data that is to be analysed. Researchers use different ways of making field notes, either written or online notes. In online research the field notes may be written notes to sketch impressions or relationships between emerging themes and concepts, or screenshots at particular time. The researcher may also make notes on certain technological features of the research setting (Salmons, 2016).

The next step is finding patterns and producing explanations using both inductive and deductive reasoning to categorise data into segments. This is known as 'coding'. A code is a symbol or abbreviation used to classify words or phrases.

Different types of codes can be used to categorise data. 'Descriptive codes' refer to how the researcher organises data and is used during the early phases of data analysis. These codes are close to the words participants used. Interpretive codes are developed further on in the process, and the name refers to looking for a deeper meaning in what the participants stated. Lastly, explanatory codes are used when the researcher starts unravelling the possible meanings, and these codes develop and even change as the researcher gains more insight about the data's meaning.

Coding and categorising are generally initiated as soon as data collection begins. Coding is used to organise data collected in interviews and other types of documents. The researcher can check the reliability of the coding by having another person encode the data and then checking for agreement. Some researchers validate findings with their participants and/or other forms of evidence. Category development is facilitated through the use of either manual or computer analysis.

Manual analysis involves a thorough review of all recorded information that the researcher has obtained during the course of data collection, including the field notes. Coding involves inventing and applying a category system. Codes that are connected conceptually are clustered into broad categories. Ideas for categories usually emerge during the coding process. For example, in the case of a participant hospitalised for six weeks and who gives an account of her perceptions of hospitalisation, the researcher could classify her statements into types of people described, feelings expressed, levels of communication, theories about communication in hospitals, activities, and so on. Thus, several codes or categories can be identified within the data recorded for any given participant. The researcher works with these categories to identify ones most prevalent, or of greatest priority for the individual. The researcher continually associates the data collected from one participant with that of another to determine a final theme.

Themes are described as abstract entities that bring identity and meaning to a current experience and its optional manifestations. The theme unifies and captures the nature of the experience into a meaningful whole. In labelling themes, a standard practice is to define the essence of each theme. A theme is not one word. That would be a topic. The theme makes a point about a topic and is always a statement. For example, in a study about stress a theme could be: 'Stress is caused by insecurity'. Another example in a study on student support during clinical placement would be: 'Suggestions to enhance clinical learning during clinical placement' or 'Support needed, identified from students' clinical learning experiences'.

Themes are never universal. In developing themes, the researcher not only attempts to discover commonalities across participants but also searches for variation. It is important then that the researcher is interested in what theme arises and in how these themes are patterned. The researcher must be sensitive to the patterns and relationships and whether the theme applies to only particular people or in certain contexts. Through integration of themes, the various thematic pieces form an integrated whole.

Rigour of the data and processes is vital. When reporting on the themes, verbatim quotes are provided to support the themes and categories. The quotes provide a link back to the original data and provide the evidence that the findings emerged from the data and that the interpretation was consistent with the experiences or perceptions of the participants. It is also good practice to have an independent coder (co-coder) to analyse the data which will enrich the rigour of the study. The researcher and the independent coder engage in a consensus-seeking discussion to reach a level of agreement on the final themes.

With the advent of computer programs, data analysis has been enhanced for qualitative researchers. The programs can sort, code and rearrange data in many ways. However, they do not completely replace or complete the data-analysis process – the researcher still must engage with it.

Data-analysis evaluation

The data-analysis portion of a research report should be carefully scrutinised to determine whether the procedures used were appropriate and correct, and whether the findings are presented meaningfully. If this is not done, there will be no satisfactory answer to the research question. An inadequate (or incorrect) analysis can produce misleading results. The researcher has an intellectual and moral responsibility to ensure quality data analysis. The following questions serve as guidelines when evaluating data-analysis strategies.

About **scientific adequacy:**
- Does the level of data measurement fit with the type of statistics used?
- Is the link between the analysis and findings logical and clear?
- Are there enough data in the form of examples, tables or graphics to allow for verification of the conclusions reached?

Concerning **statistics:**
- Are the correct and most appropriate statistics used to describe data?
- Is the statistical result presented in clear language as well as in numerical formulation?
- Is there enough evidence to verify the correctness of the statistical result?

With regard to **graphics:**

- Are the graphic displays accurate, simple and clear?
- Do they make a point without the need for a narrative?
- Do they enhance the quality of the argument, as well as the conclusions reached by the researcher?

Concerning **narrative:**

- Is the data analysis method consistent with the study's purpose?
- Are the steps in the analysing process explicitly stated?
- Have the research questions been answered?

Protection of data in the online space

A benefit of online research is the ability to easily record, save and archive the interaction or interview for further reviewing later. However, before the researcher may commence with the recording, there must be informed consent that the interview or interaction may be recorded and kept safely. Before the researcher commences with analysis of online data, it is important that all data is recorded with the permission of all those involved, including co-facilitators.

The permissions and consent related to online data could have the following detailed options:

- Permission is granted that the interview may be recorded (video and audio) and saved for purposes of the research.
- Permission is granted that audio or video clips or stills from the interview may be used as fieldnotes as well as in reports, scientific articles or academic presentations.
- Permission is clearly denied that audio or video clips or stills from the interview are used in any report or presentation.

Taking into account the above, the researcher must answer the following questions during the data analysis process on online research:

- Can I protect the data?
- What is the level of control I have over the data?
- Can I download the file and delete it from the server?
- Is there a possibility that someone can intentionally or unintentionally access the data?
- Can I allow the participants to review the recordings?
- Will I have the ability to restrict access to the recordings?
- Can I be sure that no other person can forward, download or copy the recordings?
- Will I be able to completely erase the recorded files?

If a researcher plans to use a software program to analyse the data, such as Atlas.ti., HyperResearch or NVivo, the data must be in a compatible format. In using one of these programs the same rules as in manual data analysis apply in terms of storage of the data.

Summary

In this chapter, we paid attention to data-analysis strategies, dividing the statistical methods into two broad groups. We explored the descriptive techniques and discussed frequency distributions, measures of central tendency and dispersion or variability, and correlation techniques. We briefly dealt with inferential techniques and graphics. Having touched on the analysis of qualitative data, the chapter closed with a list of the general criteria for critiquing data-analysis strategies and aspects related to the protection of online data.

Exercises

1. Students' stress levels about online practices were measured to determine their readiness to write online tests. The following scores were obtained: 41, 35, 38, 43, 29, 38, 27. Calculate the mean, median and mode.

2. A researcher studying the relationship between employees' feelings of demotivation and job satisfaction administers two inventories – one measuring job satisfaction and the other demotivation – to 100 healthcare professionals, and compares the results. The mean score on the demotivation inventory is 65.8, while the mean score on the job satisfaction inventory is 72. What statistical test should the researcher use?

3. Give an example of how standard deviation could be used in reporting an experience you have had.

4. Give an example of when a t-test should be used.

5. Rank order correlation is applied to some data, and a correlation of 0.37 is found. What does this indicate?

6. A researcher has collected data on the pulse rates and final examination marks of ten students, and would like to know if there is a relationship between the two measures. Which statistical test should be used?

7. Search for a quantitative article. Read through the analysis section and critique each test used for its suitability and application in the research.

8. Which inferential statistic would you choose for the following sets of variables? Variable 1 is whether a patient has undergone major heart surgery after a myocardial infarction. Variable 2 is whether the patient has shown signs of depressive behaviour during rehabilitation.

9. Ask eight fellow students to describe their understandings of daily revision of newly taught content, and how it affects their social life in terms of free time. Develop a coding scheme to organise the data. What major themes emerge?

10. Find a scientific article on a qualitative study. Assess whether the themes were phrased correctly. Rephrase the themes based on the discussion of the data.

11. Identify a topic for an online study. What should be included in the permission from participants in terms of the recordings of the interviews?

Research reports and report evaluation

LEARNING OUTCOMES

On completion of this chapter, you should be able to demonstrate your understanding of:

- research report formats
- the aim of a research report
- planning a research report
- how to correctly organise a research report's content
- the style and ethics of report writing
- the guidelines for critiquing a research report
- productive writing and associated factors

This chapter outlines the purpose, format, style and organisation of a research report. A research report is the document that a researcher produces as a result of a research study or investigation and summarises all the major elements of a study. It describes the study to other researchers, professionals, students or a global audience and provides the contributions that the study has made to the body of knowledge. Scientific knowledge is the sum of researchers' individual efforts – thus, clear and accurate communication of a study's results is crucial.

Purpose of a research report

A research report conveys the facts, knowledge and findings of a study as effectively as possible. The report highlights the study's essence and concludes it. It must be written in intelligible language for it to contribute to the field of interest. It is often a requirement for gaining an academic qualification or professional advancement. Dissemination of research findings is the final step of a study. Without dissemination, participants' time, data, researchers' efforts, knowledge and funding are wasted (Grove, Burns & Gray, 2013). Typical research reports contain the following elements (Polit & Beck, 2021):

- the degree to which the results are consistent with other completed research
- an interpretation of the findings and their practical significance, be it clinical or non-clinical
- implications for policy, practice and further research
- study limitations and implications for the veracity of the findings.

The aim of a research reports is therefore to answer the following questions:

- What was the study about? This is summarised in the title and abstract of the report and must therefore be concise and specific.
- How was the problem investigated?
- What has been found in this study?
- What are the implications and the meaning of the findings?
- How do these findings inform future research and practice?

Report formats

There are variations in the way in which research reports are written. They refer to the nature of the study, the purpose of the research and the report's audience. Reports are written in the form of journal articles, dissertations and theses, review reports, executive summaries and short notes.

Dissertations and theses are thorough documents (some 100 to 350 pages or more in length), which include exhaustive searches of the relevant literature. They are written in detail and in a scientific manner. By contrast, research articles and papers must demonstrate a high level of scientific quality condensed into a few pages. The average length of a journal article is between 4 000 and 6 000 words or even less. This means that the researcher must summarise the information about the study's purpose, the methods used, the findings and the interpretations in a short report. Most academic/ scientific journals have guidelines about the format and page limit of articles submitted for publication. Other research reports may include conference papers. The format of these papers is usually provided by the conference organiser and is usually much shorter, such as 1 000 words.

The format of a report is also influenced by the intended audience. For example, a report to be presented to the average educated readership (scientific community) of a journal will present the findings in contextual terms, determined by the scope and focus of the journal. It may be necessary to communicate the findings of a research study to semi-literate or illiterate people, in which case it could be presented verbally, or by using audio-visual techniques such as videotapes. This type of report must always be supported by a written report, though.

Planning the report

Planning the report is of utmost importance. It could be a daunting task to extract the most important information and present it in a limited number of words. This is especially the case where a journal article is planned from a full thesis. In such a case the researcher must compile a 5 000-word report from a 280 000-word thesis. Two categories of information can be used to compile a research report – evidence-based and non-evidence-based information (Du Plooy-Cilliers et al, 2014). Evidence-based information includes definitions, evidence and inferences, whereas non-evidence-based information entails assumptions, opinions and viewpoints. The type of report that is prepared, the audience and the scope of the publisher of the report will determine the style. Proper planning is thus of utmost importance.

When embarking of the writing process, the author must have planned properly, including the process that will be followed in preparing the report. Various models of the writing process can be found in the literature. We propose a generic model consisting of the following steps:

- Ensure you are clear about the author guidelines (in the case of a journal article or conference report) or instructions of the institution (in the case of a thesis). Make sure you understand what is expected of you. Consider what type of argument is required by the publisher. It is always helpful to read some previous publications that were approved and published in the journal or by the institution.
- Plan the structure of the report. Using a mind map or concept map may assist in ensuring that all relevant sections are covered and that word counts are divided in terms of importance or emphasis of a section. Do not start writing the report if you are not sure what should be contained in the report. If you use a mind map to plan the content of your report, this is a way to organise your ideas.
- Get started. Brainstorm ideas around the content. Add these ideas to your mind map. Sort and evaluate the ideas that were written down. Write down short notes that you think should be included. Reorganise and polish the ideas that you wrote down initially.
- Write the first draft. This will not be the only draft or version you write. Be prepared to re-write the report or sections of it more than once. Continuously keep the purpose of the report in mind. Maintain a logical flow in the argument you are conveying and present the ideas coherently. The writing may not necessarily be orderly as the structure may change. The focus is on what you want to write. Maintain a good scientific writing style and include all references right from the start. Do not think you will be able to go back and add the references; you will have difficulty in finding the correct sources for each section that you want to reference.
- Revise the draft(s) and evaluate the content critically. This step is important to improve your work. Rearrange, sift, cut, rewrite and polish the work. In this step you will inevitably identify shortcomings in what you have already written and this provides you with the opportunity to find new information or consolidate and restructure the existing content. It is also time to assess the logical flow of the argument and the presentation of information.
- Proofread the report carefully and critically. At this stage a 'critical friend' is of value. In this step you can correct any errors to ensure the report is presented professionally. The feedback from the critical reader could serve as an initial review process, allowing for improvements.
- Edit the report for grammar, spelling and punctuation. This should ideally be done by a professional editor. Ensure you adhere to the guidelines in terms of reference style.

Knowing your **audience** before you start writing is an important step in the planning phase. You could ask questions such as 'Will the audience be healthcare professionals/nurses only or will a wider audience such as educators also read the report?'; 'Will the audience be researchers or clinical practitioners who might not be involved in research?'; 'Would this article be read by members of the community who are not healthcare professionals?'; and 'Will the audience include non-English speaking persons?'

Research reports are often written with multiple audiences in mind. Planning the report must therefore include high consideration of what will be reported on and how it will be reported. It could require writing two reports with different foci, strategies, depth and content. For example, a study on the early detection and treatment of clubfoot in infants could be published in a public health journal with the focus on strategies for specialised services in rural communities to ensure early detection and treatment, thus taking the specialised services to the communities. An article could be written with a focus on midwives to provide the health education that is needed to ensure the early detection and treatment of clubfoot in infants at the antenatal and postnatal clinics.

Another matter to consider is **authorship**. This is not a problem where the report is a dissertation or thesis as there are institutional requirements. When the report is a journal article and there is more than one author, the order of the authors must be determined beforehand. Polit and Beck (2021) suggest the authorship credit and order should be based on the contribution that each author made to the research, the involvement in drafting and revising the report, approving the final report, and agreeing to be accountable for all aspects of the work. The lead author and co-authors must reach consensus about all responsibilities related to preparing, writing and finalising the report to avoid conflict. The first author (also referred to as corresponding author) is normally the lead author, but this is not essential. Ethically, it is most appropriate to list the names in the order of contribution and not according to status or post level. Where the article is based on a thesis, the student is normally the first author but might not be the lead author. Where contributions were equal, authors may decide to list the names in alphabetical order.

Structure of the report

Whatever the format, all research reports include a core of essential information. The main sections consist of the introduction, research methodology, results and findings, discussions, conclusions, recommendations and references. In addition, an abstract (which appears at the beginning), and the appendices (which appear at the end) are also included. The format of the report may, however, differ depending on the requirements of the academic institution or journal in question.

The title

The title should be an accurate reflection of the research performed and reflect its nature, population and key variables. It must be meaningful, unambiguous and brief.

Although the length of a title may vary, it should not exceed 15 words. Some authors of journal articles provide creative titles that may include an analogy or metaphor. Make sure the title is still clear and portrays the essence of the report. The reader will see the title and make a decision on whether they want to continue reading. It must therefore stimulate interest and encourage the reader to continue reading.

Abstract

The abstract must summarise the report in no more than a few short paragraphs. The number of words is determined by the publisher. It must include all elements so that the reader knows exactly what is to follow. The length of the abstract is often limited to 150 to 300 words, depending on the requirements of the publication. It should be accompanied by the most important key words (usually limited to five to ten).

Introduction to the study

Here, the research problem is introduced and the area within which the problem is situated is identified. The purpose of the study is clarified. The study's significance is emphasised, and an overview of key concepts is provided. The hypothesis, objectives or research questions are stated clearly and concisely, and logical arguments are provided to show that each statement is plausible and sound. Authoritative sources (including other scientists) are quoted to assess what is known about a particular issue and what remains unclear and requires further investigation. It is important that the introduction is particularly clear so that the reader grasps the precise nature of the study and learns about its background and context. The basic rationale and motivation for the study must be clear.

This section could be started with an interesting or controversial statement to stimulate the curiosity and interest of the reader. To assist with the logical flow of this section the author could start by providing an outline of the topic and move to an explanation of what they intend achieving and from which perspective the topic will be addressed; therefore, moving from the general to the more specific. The processes, being the approach and methodology, will be mentioned briefly.

Literature review

The literature review provides an overview of current knowledge. Both primary and secondary sources should be used. Correct referencing is important and, if not done, the researcher is guilty of plagiarism. The researcher needs to demonstrate a grasp of the theory and must also apply their knowledge to the research. Various theoretical viewpoints need to be considered. However, every aspect of the literature cannot be covered. To keep this section concise, only sources relevant to the problem are to be cited and commented upon. Indeed, only the most relevant and recent information that contributes to the argument in the study need be included. In a qualitative research report the literature will be integrated into the findings of the study as literature control rather than as an extensive review of the literature prior to data collection.

Research methodology

This section informs the reader about how the investigation was carried out, i e what the researcher did to solve the research problem or to answer the research questions. It should contain enough detail to enable another researcher to replicate the investigation and the selected methodology should be well motivated.

The research methodology section considers the population, sampling frame, approach and technique, sample size, data-collection method, and data processing and analysis, as well as strategies to enhance methodological integrity and scientific rigour. Some guidelines on how to ensure the most important information is included are listed below.

Research design and strategy

The chosen design should be specified and include the order of succession of activities, their duration and the instructions provided to participants. The choices behind strategy decisions should be outlined. The process of obtaining ethical approval and permission from the institution, as well as obtaining participants' informed consent, should be included. Strategies to enhance the methodological integrity and scientific rigour (validity, reliability and trustworthiness) should be discussed in detail.

Participants

A number of questions must be answered concerning the population and sample:

- Who, or what, constituted the population?
- Who were the participants?
- How many were there?
- How were they selected?
- Why are they appropriate for this study?
- How many participated?

Instrument and data collection

The methods used to collect data form an important component of this section. A description of all tasks or types of activities that participants were asked to perform should be described, as well as all the material and/or instruments used. For example, if participants had to fill in a questionnaire, the researcher should provide the main points of the questionnaire; if they were tested on a certain skill with a specific instrument, the researcher must describe both the instrument and the skill; if participants' reactions to a situation were observed, the researcher needs to describe in detail how this was done. The researcher must also describe the considerations which led to their choice and how validity and reliability were ensured. Specially developed devices, such as questionnaires or interview schedules, should be included in an appendix should this be indicated or allowed by the publisher.

Data analysis

The researcher must give an account of the methods and processes used for analysing the data. These depend on the nature of the research problem, objectives or questions and on the type of data. If a quantitative design was used, statistical tests applied to the obtained data are discussed. Procedures for dealing with missing data should be explained. The presentation of validity and reliability scores is important. The reasons behind the use of specific statistical tests provide meaning to the results. If a qualitative study was done, the steps of the data-analysis process to identify themes and categories (doing content analysis) must be described.

Results or findings

The main results following from the data analysis are presented, depending on the approach, design and the type of analysis undertaken. If a quantitative study was done, tables, graphs, diagrams and the outcomes of statistical tests should be used. It is essential that these representations are used carefully, and that they have precise titles and headings so that they are easily identifiable. In a quantitative study additional information is often required, eg the name of the statistical test used and the value of the calculated statistic and its significance. Accuracy and conciseness must be adhered to throughout. A good practice could be to involve a statistician as a 'critical friend' to ensure that the statistical explanations are sound.

In a qualitative study, findings are usually presented in terms of the themes which emerged from the data and, by way of substantiation and illustration, examples of raw data will be given (for instance, direct quotes from an interview transcription, or accounts of observations).

Discussion

The results are now linked to the research problem and objectives. The integration must show congruency in addressing the phenomenon under investigation. The discussion typically incorporates the following:

- an interpretation and a summary of the findings, subject to validity and reliability or trustworthiness
- conclusions related to the question(s) raised in the introduction
- integration of literature into the discussion and conclusion drawn on the main findings
- limitations identified during the study
- generalisation of the research findings, if applicable
- recommendations.

In some guidelines the conclusions, limitations and recommendations are separated. Make sure you follow the author guidelines or institutional requirements. A well-developed discussion makes sense of the results and must be presented in concise language. The researcher restates the research objectives or questions and/or hypotheses and discusses the results with reference to them in the order in which they were posed. The researcher indicates whether they found what was expected, and how the present results relate to existing research. Thus, the discussion should connect the findings with similar studies, and especially with the theory underlying them. If unexpected, inconclusive or contradictory results are obtained, possible reasons for the outcomes should be discussed.

Limitations include factors such as the inherent weakness of the sampling method, inadequate designs and controls, weaknesses in the methods used to collect data, and so forth. The researcher should identify the study's limitations and defend the validity of the findings in light of them. The researcher has the opportunity to recommend ways of minimising or eliminating the limitations, and to offer alternative methodology or improvements of the methods presented. There may be recommendations for applying the research and suggestions concerning further research.

References

The researcher must refer to the literature consulted during the study. The references should be presented in a standard manner and used consistently throughout the report. Style manuals and author guidelines should be consulted for information on how references are to be listed. The use of reference management software programs is of great help here. Sufficient information must be given to ensure that readers are able to identify and retrieve sources referred to. An entry in the reference list or bibliography should feature:

- surname(s) of the author(s) and initial(s), year of publication, title and subtitle, edition (where applicable), place of publication and publisher in the case of a **book**;
- surname(s) of the author(s) and initial(s), year, title of the article, name of journal, volume number of the relevant volume, page number(s) in the case of a **journal article**.

It is essential that every book and article cited in the text appears in the bibliography, with full details.

Style of the report

A clearly written report without unnecessary detail should be submitted. In general, the researcher should keep in mind the following:

- Avoid long phrases, pretentious words or complicated sentences. Short, simple sentences are far more easily understood.
- Use quotations sparingly. They should be used only to convey precisely the ideas of another researcher. Refer to the source, including the page number.
- Make sure that you are writing at an appropriate level for your audience.
- Make sure that you are succinct. Do not introduce issues and concepts which are not strictly relevant to reporting your investigation.
- Use an objective style.
- Organise your thoughts carefully.

The purpose of a research report is to tell the story of the study. However, not all readers may be *au fait* with all the terminology and content. Readers may struggle with the understanding for the following reasons:

- The report may be too compact and dense. Authors are usually limited to the number of pages or words allowed to explain the whole process and convey the entire 'message'.
- The terminology may seem esoteric and the jargon unfamiliar.
- Reports containing statistics (quantitative reports) may be unclear and intimidating if one does not at least have a working understanding of statistics and its meaning.
- The objectivity with which the report is written differs between quantitative and qualitative research. Quantitative reports focus on objectivity and may seem impersonal. On the other hand, qualitative research reports are written in a more conversational style.

Technical layout of the report

The technical considerations of a research report will influence the overall impression of the reader. As a scientific document, the report should include:

- A title page which contains a title, name(s) of author(s), institutional affiliations of the authors and date (month and year) of completion.
- An abstract (adhering to the number of words) and key terms.
- Numbered pages.
- A table of contents providing a complete list of headings from each part of the report, as well as relevant page numbers, where relevant.
- A list of abbreviations, acknowledgements, tables and figures (as applicable).
- A reference list for all sources used.
- Headings and subheadings organising the content and making it reader-friendly.
- A limited number of footnotes.
- Language tenses are used consistently.
- Reports are usually written in the past tense, but literature reviews may be written in the present tense.
- Language must be easily understandable.
- Use the active voice rather than the passive voice, for example: 'The fieldworker conducted focus group interviews' rather than 'Focus group interviews were conducted by the fieldworker.'
- When using abbreviations, use the full word first, with the abbreviation in brackets and thereafter the abbreviation, and be consistent.
- Use personal pronouns such as 'I' and 'we' sparingly or not at all, depending on the writing style used in the publication.
- Avoid using contractions such as 'won't' or 'can't'.
- Numbers are written in a specific style. For example:
  - Numbers up to nine, or in some cases ten, are written out in words.
  - If the sentence begins with a number, it is written as a word.
  - Statistics such as percentages, fractions or decimal figures are expressed as figures.

The ethics of report writing

Researchers have an obligation to research participants, their colleagues, their profession and the scientific community at large, to publish honest and accurate results. Attention must therefore be paid to the following:

- Data should not be invented or manipulated.
- Data or theories should not be plagiarised and reported as the researcher's original work.
- The limitations and problems of carrying out the investigation should not be concealed or ignored.
- Data should be honestly analysed and, as far as possible, interpreted without personal, political and emotional bias.

In health sciences research ethics and honesty have widespread implications. Ethics concern not only the researcher's treatment of participants but also their own competence. Poorly designed and conducted research is unethical in that it may cause harm to others.

Critical evaluation of the report

Every healthcare professional must learn how to evaluate research, even if they are not a researcher. Evaluating or critiquing a research report allows the reader to determine a study's merits and whether it is applicable to practice or the profession. No research is perfect, particularly because healthcare professionals often study people and variables in environments which are often impossible to control.

It is important for the research reader to evaluate studies objectively rather than emotionally. Leininger (1968) makes several pertinent points, still valid today, about the importance of the research critique, the role of the person doing the critique and the possible reactions of the researcher whose work is critiqued. Leininger (1968: 444) defines a research critique as 'a critical estimate of a piece of research which has been carefully and systematically studied by a critic who has used specific criteria to appraise the favourable, less favourable and other general features of the research study'. The critique should be objective, constructive and advisory, and should include the strengths, weaknesses and general features of the research being reviewed. A summary appraisal and recommendation should also be part of the critique. Leininger (1968) also believes that the research critique is a valuable and necessary means of helping a researcher to become competent in research, as well as of advancing the profession. The process of evaluating a research report requires breaking down the report into its sections and examining each of them.

Criteria designed to assist the evaluator in judging the relative value of each component of the research report follows. When undertaking a critique, the evaluator should:

- be objective

- identify positive aspects of the study and use positive terms wherever possible
- consider the report in a balanced way, that is, identify inadequacies as well as adequacies
- make comments specific to the work being reviewed and provide explanations in a constructive manner, where necessary
- explain how the study in general, the methodology and/or the findings and conclusions are relevant to the current situation or times
- discuss strengths first, then follow with points for improvement.

When undertaking a critique, the evaluator should not:

- search dogmatically for mistakes
- be petty
- focus on personal preferences
- focus on technical aspects only
- disregard the context within which the study was conducted
- try to change the study by making comments that will be regarded as 'after the fact'
- use meaningless terms such as 'bad', 'good' and 'nice'.

Common errors the evaluator should look out for are:

- insufficient or inadequate information provided in one or more components of the research process
- theoretical or conceptual frameworks which are illogical
- sentences, paragraphs or sections which may be confusing
- components which may be more complicated than necessary, as is the case when the researcher tries to combine too many theories, or to put too much into a design
- information which may be inappropriate, inapplicable or unrelated to the research question or other parts of the study
- statements which may be questionable, or supported by insufficient data or evidence
- statements which may not be supported or linked to recent and relevant data.

The first-time evaluator will understandably find critiquing difficult. It takes time and practice to develop competence. It is unrealistic for an evaluator to be skilled without practice, and delivering constructive criticism is a valuable skill. As a first-time reviewer of a journal article, the reviewer may seek assistance from a mentor.

Productive writing

Badenhorst (2010) defines **productive writing** as writing regularly, producing goal-directed reports and enjoying the process. To become a productive writer, three issues should be addressed: self-reflection, time and meaning. Self-reflection assists the researcher in determining their strengths and areas of improvement in terms of writing. Time is a crucial aspect in writing and includes planning and the motivation to get started. Meaning provides the researcher with the will to write.

The following questions may apply:

- **Why should I write or publish?** Publishing is important for all professionals, especially academics. It contributes to knowledge-building and communicating that knowledge. It is also a requirement for performance appraisal purposes and promotion in the academic context.
- **When should I write?** The best time to start is now. The researcher does not have to wait to have completed a research project to report on it. They can start by reporting on their practice and publishing in a weekly or monthly institutional newsletter or write an article for a journal which does not only publish research articles. The researcher should start writing in groups where they can share knowledge, skills and insecurities. This can be very supportive to the first-time writer. Find a writing buddy and a mentor.
- **How do I go about writing?** The writing process entails three stages. Pre-writing is the stage at which the researcher finds ideas, researches them, makes notes and draws mind maps. Questions asked in this stage are: Why am I writing? What am I writing about? What will I say? Who am I writing for? How will I say it? During the writing stage, the researcher writes to get a message across and to shape the document into the required format. The revision stage entails evaluating the writing by revising and critiquing the format, style and content, and then making the necessary changes.
- **What am I going through when writing?** When the researcher decides what they should write about, three themes can guide or block them: thinking, feeling and acting. These three are interrelated and, by pulling them together, the researcher develops text to write. Thinking is the cognitive process through which the researcher finds and processes information, and comprehends, applies, analyses, synthesises and evaluates it. Thinking entails transferring thoughts to the processes of writing, refining, structuring and revising text. Although this can be overwhelmingly complex initially, it becomes easier. We are taught that writing should be free of emotions, but feelings form an integral part of the writing process. Feelings such as anxiety, fear of rejection or failure, apprehension, joy, pleasure, worry and contentment may affect the researcher's writing and hold them hostage. Acting entails how one behaves when it comes to writing. It determines how often the researcher writes, how long the writing process takes them, which strategies they use to start writing, what stops them from writing and finishing what they started, and how and/or why they avoid writing.

Once the researcher has decided to start writing, they should ask themselves these questions and answer them honestly. By changing our perceptions, we can control the way we understand ourselves in terms of the ability and willingness to write. Motivation is the reason we decide to do something. Through thinking, feeling and acting, the researcher can get the process started.

Productive writing facilitates a good report. Follow-up reports in the form of articles should also be part of the healthcare professional's research role.

Summary

In this chapter, we outlined the general format that a researcher must follow when writing up study results. We emphasised the responsibility that the researcher has to use a clear, comprehensive and accurate style to facilitate readers' understanding, or so that other researchers can replicate the project. The researcher is also ethically bound, we pointed out, to report the findings in an unbiased and truthful manner. Lastly, we explored aspects of the critical evaluation of a research report and of productive writing.

Exercises

1. Debate the importance of disseminating research findings to the scientific community. Also consider the value of dissemination for knowledge translation.

2. Select a topic and search for articles using one of the electronic search engines. Choose five articles based on their titles and justify why the titles drew your attention.

3. Select two or three research articles. Identify the key elements of each.

4. Select another research article and evaluate it using the criteria outlined in this chapter.

5. As a novice author or researcher, what are your biggest fears when thinking about writing a research report?

6. In the section of the report entitled 'Discussion', what does the writer inform the readers about?

7. Identify three journals in which you could present a report. Read the guidelines to authors, and compare the similarities and differences of the requirements.

8. Read the section on productive writing in this chapter again and relate it to your own experiences. How will they affect you when you are required to write an article?

Bibliography

Ader, HJ and Mellenbergh, GJ. 1999. Research Methodology in the Social, Behavioural and Life Sciences. London: SAGE Publications.

Ahrens, EH. 1992. The Crisis in Clinical Research. New York: Oxford University Press.

Alien, JD. 1989. Women who successfully manage their weight. Western Journal of Nursing Research 11(6): 657–75.

Altman, DG. n.d. Statistics and Ethics in Medical Research. Harrow, Middlesex: Clinical Research Centre.

Alvesson, Mats, and Jorgen Sandberg. 2001. Re-imagining the Research Process. SAGE Publications, Ltd. (UK).

Arminger, B. 1977. Ethics of nursing research: Profile, principles, perspective. Nursing Research 26(5): 330–6.

Babbie, E and Mouton, J. 2021. The Practice of Social Research. 15th ed. Cape Town: Oxford University Press.

Badenhorst, C. 2010. Productive Writing: Becoming a Prolific Academic Writer. Pretoria: Van Schaik.

Bergman, MM. 2010. On Concepts and Paradigms in Mixed Methods Research. Journal of Mixed Methods Research 4(3): 171–175.

Birks, M & Mills, J. 2011. Grounded Theory: A Practical Guide. Los Angeles: SAGE Publications.

Bless, C, Higson-Smith, C and Sithole, SL. 2013. Fundamentals of Social Research Methods: An African Perspective 5th ed. Cape Town: Juta.

Booysen, S. 2003. Designing a questionnaire. In Intellectual Tools: Skills for the Human Sciences 2nd ed, ed D Rossouw. Pretoria: Van Schaik.

Boswell, C and Cannon, S. 2007. Introduction to Nursing Research: Incorporating Evidence-based Practice. Boston: Jones and Bartlett.

Botes, A. 2003. Validity, reliability and trustworthiness. In Intellectual Tools: Skills for the Human Sciences 2nd ed, ed D Rossouw. Pretoria: Van Schaik.

Botma, Y, Greeff, M, Mulaudzi, FM and Wright, SCD. 2010. Research in Health Sciences. Cape Town: Heinemann.

Bowling, A. 2002. Research Methods in Health: Investigating Health and Services 2nd ed. Berkshire: Open University Press.

Bowling, A and Ebrahim, S (eds). 2005. Handbook of Health Research Methods. New York: McGraw-Hill Education.

Breakwell, GM, Hammond, S and Fife-Schaw, C. 2000. Research Methods in Psychology 2nd ed. London: SAGE Publications.

Brink, PJ and Wood, MJ. 1998. Advanced Design in Nursing Research 2nd ed. London: SAGE Publications.

Brink, PJ and Wood, MJ. 1999. Basic Steps in Planning Nursing Research. Boston: Jones and Bartlett.

Brockopp, DY and Hastings-Tolsma, MX. 1995. Fundamentals of Nursing Research. Boston: Jones and Bartlett.

Brown, B, Crawford, P and Hicks, C. 2003. Evidence-based Research: Dilemmas and Debates in Health Care. Berkshire: Open University Press.

Brunger, F, Russel, T and Wall, D. 2021. Decolonizing Research Ethics: Best Practices for the Ethical Conduct of Research Involving Indigenous Peoples. Scholarly Research Reviews. Oxford Handbooks Online.

Burns, N and Grove, SK. 2020. The Practice of Nursing Research: Appraisal, synthesis and generation of evidence. 9th ed. Philadelphia: Elsevier.

Burns, N and Grove, SK. 2019. Understanding Nursing Research: Building an evidence-based practice 7th ed. Philadelphia: Saunders.

Campbell, D and Stanley, J. 1966. Experimental and Quasi-experimental Designs for Research. Chicago: Rand McNally.

Charmaz, K. 2014. Constructing Grounded Theory 2nd ed. Los Angeles: SAGE Publications.

Chenitz, WC and Swanson, JM. 1986. From Practice to Grounded Theory: Qualitative Research in Nursing. Menlo Park: Addison-Wesley.

Chinn, PL and Kramer, MK. 1999. Theory and Nursing: A Systematic Approach. St Louis: Mosby.

Chinn, PL and Kramer, MK. 2011. Integrated Theory and Knowledge Development in Nursing 8th ed. St Louis: Elsevier Mosby.

Chinn, PL and Kramer, MK. 2015. Knowledge Development in Nursing: Theory and Process 9th ed. St Louis: Elsevier Mosby.

Clare, J and Hamilton, H. 2003. Writing Research: Transforming Data into Text. Edinburgh: Churchill Livingstone.

Clark, T, Foster, L, Sloan, L and Bryman, A. 2021. Bryman's Social Research Methods 6th ed. Oxford: Oxford University Press.

Clifford, CL and Clark, J (eds). 2004. Getting Research into Practice. Edinburgh: Churchill Livingstone.

Cohen, J. 1977. Statistical Power Analysis for the Behavioural Sciences. New York: Academic Press.

Collaizi, PF. 1978. Psychological research as the phenomenologist views it. In Existential Phenomenological Alternatives for Psychology, eds R Valle and M King. New York: Oxford University Press.

Corbin, J and Strauss, A. 2008. Basics of Qualitative Research 3rd ed. Thousand Oaks: SAGE Publications.

Cormack, DPS. 1991. The Research Process in Nursing 2nd ed. Oxford: Blackwell Science.

Craig, JV and Smyth, RL. 2007. The Evidence-based Practice Manual for Nurses 2nd ed. London: Elsener.

Creamer, E 2018. In introduction to fully integrated mixed methods research. Thousand Oaks, CA: Sage Publications.

Creswell, JW. 2014. Qualitative Inquiry & Research Design: Choosing among Five Approaches 4th ed. Los Angeles: SAGE Publications.

Creswell JW and Creswell JD. 2018. Research Design: Quantitative, Qualitative & Mixed Method Approaches. 5th Edition. Thousand Oaks: Sage Publishers

Creswell, JW and Plano Clark, VL. 2018. Designing and conducting mixed methods research. 3rd ed. Thousand Oaks, CA: Sage Publications.

Deliktas, A., Korukcu, O., Aydin, R., and Kabukcuoglu, K. (2019). Nursing Students' Perceptions of Nursing Metaparadigms: A Phenomenological Study. The journal of nursing research : JNR, 27(5), e45. https://doi.org/10.1097/jnr.0000000000000311

Denscombe, M. 2010. The good research guide for small scale social research projects. 4th ed. Open University Press: McGraw-Hill Education.

Department of Health. 2015. Ethics in Health Research: Principles, processes and structures. 2nd ed. Republic of South Africa.

Declaration of Helsinki. 1946. In Philosophical Medical Ethics, R Gillan. Chichester: Wiley.

Denzin, NK. 1989. Interpretive Interactionism. Newbury Park: SAGE Publications.

Dickhoff, J and James, P. 1968. A theory of theories: A position paper. Nursing Research 17(3): 197–203.

Du Plooy-Cilliers, F, Davis, C and Bezuidenhout, R. 2014. Research matters. Cape Town: Juta.

Dubin, R. 1978. Theory Building rev ed. New York: Free Press.

Ellis, P. 2019. Evidence-Based Practice in Nursing 4th ed. London: Sage.

Ellis, Peter. 2022. Understanding Research for Nursing Students. 5th ed. SAGE Publications, Ltd. (UK).

Fawcett, J. 1989. Analysis and Evaluation of Conceptual Models of Nursing. Philadelphia: Aspen.

Fawcett, J and Downs, F. 1986. The Relationship of Theory and Research. Norwalk: Appleton-Century-Crofts.

Feyerabend, P. 1975. Against Method. London: Verso.

Field, PA and Morse, JM. 1985. Nursing Research: The Application of Qualitative Approaches. Kent: Croome Helm.

Fink, A. 2008. Practicing Research: Discovering Evidence that Matters. Thousand Oaks: SAGE Publications.

Flick, U. 2014. An introduction to qualitative research. London: SAGE Publications.

Garbers, JG (ed). 1996. Effective Research in the Human Sciences. Pretoria: Van Schaik.

Giorgi, A. 1970. Psychology as a Human Science. New York: Harper and Row.

Giovanetti, P. 1981. Sampling techniques. In Research Methodology and its Application to Nursing, ed YM Williamson, 169–90. New York: Wiley.

Glaser, B and Strauss, A. 1967. The Discovery of Grounded Theory: Strategies for Qualitative Research. Chicago: Aldine.

Gray, DE. Doing Research in the Real World., 5th ed. SAGE Publications, Ltd. (UK), 2021.

Gray, J, Grove, SK and Sutherland, S. 2017. The Practice of Nursing Research: Appraisal, Synthesis and Generation of Evidence 8th ed. Mosby: Elsevier.

Green, J and Thorogood, N. 2009. Qualitative Methods for Health Research. London: SAGE Publications.

Grove, SK, Burns, N and Gray, JR 2013. The Practice of Nursing Research: Appraisal, Synthesis and Generation of Evidence 7th ed. Elsevier.

Grove, SK, Gray, JR and Burns, N. 2018. Understanding Nursing Research: Building an Evidence-based Practice. 7th ed. Elsevier.

Guba, EY. 1990. The Paradigm Dialogue. Newbury Park: SAGE Publications.

Guba, E and Lincoln, Y. 1994. Competing paradigms in qualitative research. Thousand Oaks: SAGE.

Harkness, GA. 1995. Epidemiology in Nursing Practice. St Louis: Mosby.

Harvey, M& Land, L. 2021. Research Methods for Nurses and Midwives. Available from: VitalSource Bookshelf, 2nd ed. SAGE Publications, Ltd. (UK).

Hastings, J (ed). 1961. Encyclopedia of Religion and Ethics. New York: Scribner.

Hesse-Biber, SN and Johnson, RB. 2015. The Oxford Handbook of Multimethod and Mixed Methods Research Inquiry. Oxford University Press.

Hinds, PS, Scandrett-Hibden, S and McAulay, LS. 1990. Further assessment of a method to estimate reliability and validity of qualitative research findings. Journal of Advanced Nursing 15(4): 430–5.

Hockey, L. 1991. The nature and purpose of research. In The Research Process in Health Care Sciences, ed DPS Cormack. London: Blackwell Science.

Houser, J. 2008. Nursing Research: Reading, Using, and Creating Evidence. Boston: Jones and Bartlett.

Human Sciences Research Council (HSRC). n.d. Research Code. Pretoria: HSRC.

Hutchison, J. 1977. Living Options in World Philosophy. Honolulu: University Press of Hawaii.

International Council of Nurses (ICN). 1996. Ethical Guidelines for Nursing Research. Geneva: ICN.

Joanna Briggs Institute. 2011. Levels of evidence FAME. http://www.joannabriggs.edu. au/ (Accessed 24 October 2011).

Jooste, K (ed). 2022. Principles and Practice of Nursing and Healthcare. 2nd ed. Pretoria: Van Schaik.

King, IM. 1981. A Theory for Nursing Systems, Concepts, Process. New York: Wiley.

Kirk, J and Miller, ML. 1986. Reliability and Validity in Qualitative Research. Beverley Hills: SAGE Publications.

Kuhn, TS. 1970. The Structure of Scientific Revolutions 2nd ed. Chicago: University of Chicago Press.

Kuhn, TS. 1977. Second thoughts on paradigms. In The Structure of Scientific Theory, edited by F Suppe, 459–82. Urbana: University of Illinois Press.

Lancaster, W and Lancaster, J. 1981. Models and model building in nursing. Advances in Nursing Science 3(3): 31–42.

Laudan, L. 1977. Progress and its Problems: Toward a Theory of Scientific Growth. Berkeley: University of California.

Laudan, L. 1995. Beyond Positivism and Relativism: Theory, method and evidence. Boulder: Westview Press.

Le Compte, MD and Goetz, JP. 1982. Problems of reliability and validity in ethnographic research. Review of Educational Research 52(1): 31–60.

Leavy, P. 2017. Research design. London: The Guilford Press.

Leedy, PD and Ormrod, JE. 2010. Practical Research: Planning and Design 9th ed. Boston: Pearson Education.

Leeman, J, Voils, CI and Sandelowski, M. 2016. Conducting Mixed Methods Literature Reviews: Synthesizing the Evidence Needed to Develop and Implement Complex Social and Health Interventions. Oxford Library of Psychology. https://doi.org/10.1093/oxfordhb/9780199933624.013.12

Leininger, MM. 1968. The research critique: Nature, function and act. Nursing Research 17(5): 444–9.

Leininger, MM (ed). 1985. Qualitative Research Methods in Nursing. Orlando: Grune and Gratton.

Leininger, MM. 1991. Transcultural care principles, human rights, and ethical considerations. Journal of Transcultural Nursing 3(1): 21–23.

Lincoln, Y and Guba, E. 1985. Naturalistic Enquiry. Beverley Hills, CA: SAGE Publications.

LoBiondo-Wood, G and Haber, J. 2010. Nursing Research: Methods and Critical Appraisal for Evidence-based Practice. St Louis: Mosby.

LoBiondo-Wood, G and Haber, J. 2014. Nursing Research: Text and Study Package 8th ed. London: Elsevier.

Machi, LA and McEvoy, BT. 2016. The literature review: six steps to success. 3rd ed. London: SAGE Publication.

Maree, JG (ed). 2016. First Steps in Research 2nd ed. Pretoria: Van Schaik Publishers.

Marriner, A. 1986. Nursing Theorists and their Work. St Louis: Mosby.

Masterman, M. 1970. The nature of a paradigm. In Criticism and the Growth of Knowledge, eds I Lakatos and A Musgrave. Cambridge: Cambridge University Press.

Medical Research Council (MRC). 2004. Guidelines on Ethics for Medical Research: General Principles 4th ed. Pretoria: MRC.

Mehmetoglu, Mehmet, and Matthias Mittner. Applied Statistics Using R. SAGE Publications, Ltd. (UK), 2021.

Meleis, A. 1985. Theoretical Nursing: Development and Progress. Philadelphia: Lippincott.

Merton, R. 1968. Social Theory and Social Structure. New York: Free Press.

Miles, MB, Huberman, AM and Saldana, J. 2013. Qualitative Data Analysis: A Methods Sourcebook. Thousand Oaks: SAGE Publications.

Mitchell, AJ. 2018. A Review of Mixed Methods, Pragmatism and Abduction Techniques. The Electronic Journal of Business Research Methods, 16(3): 103–116.

Moody, L, Vera, H, Blanks, C and Visscher, M. 1989. Developing questions of substance for nursing science. Western Journal of Nursing Research II: 392–403.

Moody, LE. 1990. Advancing Nursing Science through Research Vol 1. Newbury Park: SAGE Publications.

Morse, JM (ed). 2016. Establishing Rigor in Qualitative Inquiry. Newbury Park: SAGE Publications.

Mouton, J. 2002. Understanding Social Research. Pretoria: Van Schaik.

Muir Gray, JA. 1997. Evidence-based Health Care: How to Make Health Policy and Management Decisions. New York: Churchill Livingstone.

Muller, ME and Bester, P. 2016. Nursing Dynamics. 5th ed. Johannesburg: Pearson.

Munhall, PL. 2001. Nursing Research – A Qualitative Perspective 3rd ed. Boston: Jones and Bartlett.

Neuman, WL. 2003. Social Research Methods: Qualitative and Quantitative Approaches 5th ed. USA: Pearson Education.

Newhouse, RP, Dearholt, SL, Poe, SS, Pugh, LC and White, KM. 2007. Johns Hopkins Nursing Evidence-based Practice Model and Guidelines. Indianapolis: STTI.

Newman, M. 1983. Theory Development in Nursing. Philadelphia: Davis.

Nieswiadomy, R. 2012. Foundations of Nursing Research. 6th ed. Norwalk: Appleton and Lange.

NIH (National Institutes of Health). 2004. World Medical Association Declaration of Helsinki. http://ohsr.od.nih.gov/guidelines/helsinki.html (Accessed 25 October 2011).

Nuremberg Code. 1990. In Nursing Ethics through the Lifespan, FL Bandman and B Bandman. Norwalk: Appleton and Lange.

Orem, D. 1985. Concepts of Practice 3rd ed. New York: McGraw-Hill.

Ornery, A. 1988. Ethnography. In Paths to Knowledge, ed B Sarter. New York: National League for Nursing.

Owen, BD. 1989. The magnitude of low-back problems in nursing. Western Journal of Nursing Research 11(2): 234–42.

Padgett, DK. 2017. Qualitative Methods in Social Work Research 3rd ed. Los Angeles: SAGE Publications.

Palmer, I. 1977. Florence Nightingale: Reformer, reactionary, researcher. Nursing Research 26(2): 84–9.

Parse, RR. 1987. Nursing Science: Major Paradigms, Theories and Critiques. Philadelphia: Saunders.

Parse, RR. 2014. The Humanbecoming Paradigm: A Transformational Worldview. Pittsburgh: Discovery International Publication.

Polgar, S and Thomas, SA. 2000. Introduction to Research in the Health Sciences 4th ed. Edinburgh: Churchill Livingstone.

Polit, DF and Beck, CT. 2022. Essentials of Nursing Research: Appraising evidence for nursing practice 10th ed. Wolters Kluwer.

Polit, DF, and Beck, CT. 2021. Nursing Research: Generating and Assessing Evidence for Nursing Practice 11th ed. Philadelphia: Lippincott Williams & Wilkins.

Polit, DF, and Beck, CT. 2004. Nursing Research: Principles and methods. 7th ed. Philadelphia: Lippincott Williams & Wilkins.

Proctor, S and Renfrew, M (eds). 2001. Linking Research and Practice in Midwifery: A Guide to Evidence-based Practice. Edinburgh: Baillière Tindall.

Republic of South Africa. 2015. Ethics in Health Research: Principles, Processes and Structures. Department of Health. http://www.sun.ac.za/english/research-innovation/Research- Development/Documents (Accessed 10 March 2022).

Riemen, DJ. 1986. The essential structure of a caring interaction: Doing phenomenology. In Nursing Research: A Qualitative Perspective, eds PL Munhall and CJ Oiler. Norwalk: Appleton-Century-Crofts.

Roestenburg, WJH, Strydom, H, Fouché, CB and De Vos, AS. 2021. Research at Grass Roots: For the Social Sciences and Human Services Professions 5th ed. Pretoria: Van Schaik.

Rogers, ME. 1970. An Introduction to the Theoretical Basis of Nursing. Philadelphia: Davis.

Rossouw, D (ed). 2003. Intellectual Tools: Skills for the Human Sciences 2nd ed. Pretoria: Van Schaik.

Roy, C. 1984. Introduction to Nursing: An Adaptation Model 2nd ed. Englewood Cliffs: Prentice Hall.

Russell, B. 1945. A History of Western Philosophy. New York: Simon and Schuster.

Sackett, DL, Strauss, SE, Richardson, WS et al. 2000. Evidence-based Medicine 2nd ed. Edinburgh: Churchill Livingstone.

Salmons, J. 2016. Doing qualitative research online. London: Sage

Saunders, H. and Vehviläinen-Julkunen, K. 2016. The state of readiness for evidence-based practice among nurses: an integrative review. International Journal of Nursing Studies, 56: 128–140.

Searle, C. 1990. Research as a modifier of the constraints in developing nursing practice in South Africa: An overview. In Nursing Research for Nursing Practice: An International Perspective, ed R Bergman. London: Chapman and Hall.

Sheppard, M. 2004. Appraising and Using Social Research in the Human Services: An Introduction for Social Work and Health Professionals. London: Jessica Kingsley Publishers.

Simmons, LW and Henderson, V. 1964. Nursing Research: A Survey and Assessment. New York: Appleton-Century-Crofts.

South African Medical Research Council (MRC). 2022. Research Integrity and Responsible Conduct of Research. https://www.samrc.ac.za/research/ethics/guideline-documents.

Spradley, J. 1980. Participant Observation. New York: Holt, Rinehart and Winston.

Stake, RE. 2003. Case studies. In Strategies of Qualitative Inquiry 2nd ed, eds NK Denzin and YS Lincoln. Thousand Oaks: SAGE Publications.

Stewart, DW and Shamdasani, PN. 2015. Focus Groups: Theory and Practice. Los Angeles: SAGE Publications.

Streubert, HJ and Carpenter, DR. 2011. Qualitative Research in Nursing: Advancing the Humanistic Imperative 5th ed. Philadelphia: Lippincott Williams & Wilkens.

Struwig, FW and Stead, GB. 2001. Planning, Designing and Reporting Research. Cape Town: Pearson Education.

Tashakkori, A and Teddlie, C. 2010. SAGE Handbook of Mixed Methods in Social & Behavioral Research. 2nd ed. London: SAGE Publications.

Terre Blanche, M, Durrheim, K and Painter, D. 2016. Research in practice. 2nd ed. Cape Town: UCT Press.

Tesch, R. 1990. Qualitative research: analysis types and software tools. New York: Falmer.

Tesch, R. 1991. Computer programs that assist in the analysis of qualitative data: An overview. Qualitative Health Research 1(3): 309–25.

Thomas, R. 2019. Little quick fix: Turn your literature review into an argument. London: SAGE Publications.

Trinder, L and Reynolds, S (eds). 2001. Evidence-based Practice: A Critical Appraisal. Oxford: Blackwell Science.

Van Manen, M. 1990. Researching Lived Experiences. New York: State University of New York.

Walker, LO and Avant, KG. 2010. Strategies for Theory Construction in Nursing 4th ed. Upper Saddle River: Prentice Hall.

Watson J. 2008. Nursing: The philosophy and science of caring (Revised ed.). Louisville, CO: University Press of Colorado.

Watson. 2021. Caring Science as sacred science. New revised edition. Lotus Library: Watson Caring Science Institute.

Webb, P, Bain, C and Pirozzo, S. 2005. Essential Epidemiology: An Introduction for Students and Health Professionals. Cambridge: Cambridge University Press.

Wilson, V. 2014. Research Methods: Sampling. Evidence Based Library and Information Practice 9(2). https://journals.library.ualberta.ca/eblip/index.php/EBLIP/article/view/22186/16560 (Accessed 23 August 2017).

Woods, NF and Catanzaro, M. 1988. Nursing Research: Theory and Practice. St Louis: Mosby.

World Medical Association. 1964. Human Experimentation Code of Ethics of the World Medical Association. Declaration of Helsinki. British Medical Journal (2): 177.

Glossary

A

abduction Focuses on theory generation or modification by integrating existing theory where suitable, to build new theory or adapt existing theory

abstracts (research abstracts) Brief summaries of research studies, which generally contain the purpose, methods and major findings of the study. The abstract usually precedes the study report.

accessible population The group of people or objects that is available to the researcher for a particular study.

adequacy A desirable attribute of sampling whereby sufficient numbers of participants (or objects) have been sampled to represent the population accurately.

acquiescence response set A type of response set bias in which a participant may have a tendency to answer 'yes' or to agree with the content of the questions.

ambiguous questions Questions that contain words that may be interpreted in more than one way.

anonymity The identity of research participants is unknown, even to the study investigator(s).

applied research Research that is conducted to find a solution to an immediate, practical problem.

assent the affirmative agreement of a vulnerable individual, such as a child, to participate in a study to supplement the formal consent by a parent or legal guardian.

assumptions Basic ideas that are held to be true, but have not necessarily been proven. Assumptions may be explicit or implicit.

attitude scales Self-report data-collection instruments that ask respondents to report their attitudes or feelings on a continuum.

attribute variables – *see* demographic variables.

B

bar graph A figure used to represent a frequency distribution of nominal or ordinal data.

basic research (pure research) Research that is conducted to generate knowledge rather than to solve immediate problems.

bias Any influence that produces a distortion in the results of a study or that strongly favours the outcome of a particular finding of a research study.

bimodal A frequency distribution that contains two identical high-frequency values.

bivariate study A research study in which the relationship between two variables is examined.

bracketing In qualitative data analysis, this is the process of putting aside what is known about a study topic to allow the data to convey undistorted information.

C

cells Boxes in a table that are formed by the intersection of rows and columns.

chi-square test (x2) A non-parametric statistical test that is used to compare sets of data that are in the form of frequencies or percentages (nominal level data).

class interval A group of scores in a frequency distribution.

clinical research These kinds of studies involve clients or study alternatives.

closed-ended questions Questions that require respondents to choose from given alternatives.

cluster random sampling A random sampling process that involves two or more stages. The population is first listed by clusters or categories (for example, hospitals), and then the sample elements (for example, hospital administrators) are randomly selected from these clusters.

cohort study A special type of longitudinal study in which participants have been born during one particular period or who have similar backgrounds.

collectively exhaustive categories Categories that are provided for every possible answer.

columns Vertical entries in a table.

comparative studies Studies in which intact groups are compared on some dependent variable. The researcher is not able to manipulate the independent variable, which is frequently some inherent characteristic of the participants, such as age or educational level.

comparison group The group of participants in an experimental study that do not receive any experimental treatment, or receive an alternative treatment such as the 'normal' or routine treatment. (*See* control group.)

computer-assisted literature searches The use of a computer to obtain bibliographic references that have been stored in a database.

concept A word picture or mental idea stored in a database.

conceptual framework The background or information for a study; a less well-developed structure than a theoretical framework. Concepts are related in a logical manner by the researcher.

conceptual model Symbolic presentation of concepts and the relationships between these concepts.

concurrent validity A type of criterion validity of an instrument in which a determination is made of the instrument's ability to obtain a measurement of participants' behaviour that is comparable to some other criterion used to indicate that behaviour.

confidence interval A range of values that, with a specified degree of probability, is thought to contain the population value.

confidentiality The identity of the research participants is known only to the study investigator(s).

construct A highly abstract phenomenon that cannot be directly observed, but must be inferred by certain concrete or less abstract indicators of the phenomenon.

construct validity The ability of an instrument to measure the construct that it is intended to measure.

content analysis A data-analysis method that examines communication messages that are usually in written form.

content validity The degree to which an instrument covers the scope and range of information that is sought.

contingency table A table that visually displays the relationship between sets of nominal data.

control group A group of participants in an experimental study that do not receive the experimental treatment. (*See* comparison group.)

convenience sampling (accidental samplings) A non-probability sampling procedure that involves the selection of the most readily available people or objects for a study.

correlation The extent to which values of one variable (X) are related to the values of a second variable (Y). Correlations can be either positive or negative.

correlation coefficient A statistic that represents the magnitude and direction of a relationship between two variables. Correlation coefficients range from −1.00 (perfect negative relationship) to +1.00 (perfect positive relationship).

correlation studies Research studies that examine the strength of relationships between variables.

correlation validity The extent to which an instrument corresponds or correlates with some criterion measure of the information that is being sought; the ability of an instrument to determine participants' responses at present or predict participants' responses in the future.

critical region (region of rejection) An area in a theoretical sampling distribution that contains the critical values, or values that are considered to be statistically significant.

critical value A scientific cut-off point that denotes the value in a theoretical distribution at which all obtained values from a sample that are equal to or beyond that point are said to be statistically significant.

critique Analytical examination of a research report or proposal that involves a systematic assessment based on accepted standards of enquiry and communication.

cross-sectional study A research study that collects data on participants at one point in time.

D

data The pieces of information or facts collected during a research study.

deductive reasoning A reasoning process that proceeds from the general to the specific, from theory to empirical data.

degrees of freedom (df) A concept in inferential statistics that concerns the number of values that are free to vary.

Delphi technique A data-collection method that uses several rounds of questions to seek a consensus on a particular topic from a group of experts on the topic.

demographic questions Questions that gather data on characteristics of the participants. (*See* demographic variables.)

demographic variables Participant characteristics such as age, educational levels and marital status.

dependent variable The 'effect'; the variable that is influenced by the independent variable.

descriptive statistics The statistics that organise and summarise the numerical data obtained from populations and samples.

descriptive studies Research studies in which phenomena are described, or the relationship between variables is examined; no attempt is made to determine cause-and-effect relationships.

double-barrelled questions Questions that ask two questions in one.

E

element A single member of a population.

empirical data Objective data gathered through the sense organs.

empirical generalisation A summary statement about the occurrence of phenomena that is based on empirical data from a number of research studies.

equivalence reliability The degree to which two forms of an instrument obtain the same results, or to which two or more observers obtain the same results when using a single instrument to measure a variable.

ethnographic studies Research studies that involve the collection and analysis of data about cultural groups.

evidence-based practice The integration of best research evidence with clinical expertise and patient values.

experimenter effect A threat to the internal validity of a research study that occurs when the researcher's behaviour influences the participants' behaviour in a way that is not intended by the researcher.

explanatory studies Research studies that are conducted when little is known about the phenomenon that is being studied.

***ex post facto* studies** Studies in which the variation on the dependent variable has already occurred in the past, and the researcher is trying to determine, 'after the fact', if the variation that has occurred in the independent variable has any influence on the dependent variable that is being measured in the present.

external criticism (external appraisal, external examination) A type of examination of historical data that is concerned with the authenticity or genuineness of the data. External criticism would be used to determine if a letter was actually written by the person whose signature was evident on the letter.

external validity The degree to which study results can be generalised to other people and other research settings.

extraneous variable (intervening variable, confounding variable) A type of variable that is not the variable of interest to a researcher but that may influence the results of a study.

F

face validity A subjective determination that an instrument is adequate for obtaining the desired information; on the surface, or on the 'face' of it, the instrument appears to be an adequate means of obtaining the desired data.

field studies Research studies that are conducted 'in the field' or in a real-life setting.

filler questions Questions used to distract respondents from the purpose of other questions that are being asked.

frequency counts The listing or counting of each observation in a category; appropriate for nominal and ordinal data.

frequency polygon A graph that uses dots connected with straight lines to represent the frequency distribution of interval or ratio data A dot is placed above the midpoint of each class interval.

G

grounded theory studies Research studies in which first data are collected and analysed, and then a theory is developed that is 'grounded' in the data.

H

Hawthorne effect A threat to the internal validity of a research study that occurs when study participants respond in a certain manner because they are aware that they are involved in a research study.

health sciences research A systematic, objective process of analysing phenomena of importance to health scientists.

high risk Where there is direct human participant involvement. A real or foreseeable risk of harm including physical, psychological and social risk that may lead to a serious adverse event if not managed responsibly.

histogram A graph used to represent the frequency distribution of variables measured at the interval or ratio level.

historical studies Research studies that are concerned with the identification, location, evaluation and synthesis of data from the past.

history A threat to the internal validity of an experimental research study; some event besides the experimental treatment occurs between the pre-treatment and post-treatment measurement of the dependent variable, and this event influences the dependent variable.

hypothesis A statement of the predicted relationship between two or more variables.

I

independent variable The cause or the variable that is sought to influence the dependent variable; in experimental research it is the variable that is manipulated by the researcher.

indexes Compilations of reference materials that provide information on books and periodicals.

inductive reasoning A reasoning process that proceeds from the specific to the general, from empirical data to theory.

inferential statistics The group of statistics that is concerned with the characteristics of populations and that uses sample data to make an inference about the population.

informed consent A participant voluntarily agrees to participate in a research study in which he/she has full understanding of the study before the study begins.

interaction effect The result of two variables acting in conjunction.

internal criticism A type of examination of historical data that is concerned with the accuracy of the data. Internal criticism would be used to determine if a document contained an accurate recording of events as these actually happened.

internal validity The degree to which changes in the dependent variable (effect) can be attributed to the independent or experimental variable (cause).

interobserver reliability *See* interrater reliability.

interrater reliability (interobserver reliability) The degree to which two or more independent judges are in agreement about ratings or observations of events or behaviours.

interval level of measurement Data can be categorised and ranked, and the distance between the ranks can be specified. There is no absolute zero level. Temperature readings are examples of interval data.

interview A method of data collection in which the interviewer obtains responses from a participant in a face-to-face encounter or through a telephone call.

interview schedule An instrument containing a set of questions, directions for asking those questions and space to record the respondents' answers.

K

knowledge translation Assessment, review, and utilisation of scientific research to address the gap between the large volume of research data and its systematic review and implementation by key stakeholders. It is both a process and a strategy that could lead to utilisation of research findings and improved outcomes for consumers, students and patients.

L

laboratory studies Research studies in which participants are studied in a

special environment that has been created and controlled by the researcher.

Likert scale An attitude scale named after its developer, Renis Likert. These scales usually contain five or seven responses for each item, ranging from 'strongly agree' to 'strongly disagree'.

limitations Weaknesses in a study; uncontrolled variables.

longitudinal study Participants are followed during a period in the future and data are collected at two or more time periods.

low risk Where there is direct human participant involvement. The only foreseeable risk of harm is the potential for minor discomfort or inconvenience, thus research that would not pose a risk above the everyday norm.

M

manipulation The independent or experimental variable is controlled by the researcher to determine its effect on the dependent variable.

maturation A threat to the internal validity of an experimental research study that occurs when changes take place within study participants as a result of the passage of time (growing older, taller) and these changes may affect the study results.

medium risk Where there is direct human participant involvement. Research that poses a risk above the everyday norm, including physical, psychological and social risks. Steps can be taken to minimise the likelihood of the event occurring.

methodological studies Research studies that are concerned with the development, testing and evaluation of research instruments and methods.

mixed methods designs Designs where both qualitative and quantitative approaches are used in different order and varying levels of dominance and order. It includes at least one quantitative and one qualitative method that embrace incompatible assumptions about the nature of the world and allow researchers to mix epistemologies.

mortality A threat to the internal validity of an experimental research study that occurs when participant drop-out rate is different between the experimental group and the comparison group.

multimodal A frequency distribution in which more than two values have the same high frequency.

mutually exclusive categories Categories are uniquely distinct; no overlap occurs between categories.

N

negative relationship (inverse relationship) A relationship between two variables in which there is a tendency for the values of one variable to increase as the values of the other variable decrease.

negatively skewed A frequency distribution in which the tail of the distribution points to the left.

negligible risk Where there is no or indirect human participant involvement.

nominal level of measurement The lowest level of measurement; data are 'named' or categorised, such as race and marital status.

non-directional research hypothesis A type of research hypothesis in which a prediction is made that a relationship exists between variables, but the type of relationship is not specified.

non-equivalent control group design A type of quasi-experimental design, similar to the pre-test–post-test control group experimental design, with the exception of random assignment of participants to groups.

non-parametric tests (distribution-free statistics) A type of inferential statistics that is not concerned with population parameters; requirements for their use are less stringent and they can be used with nominal and ordinal data and small sample sizes.

non-participant observer – overt The researcher openly states that he/she is conducting research and provides participants with information about the type of data that will be collected.

non-probability sampling (including convenience, quota and purposive sampling) A sampling process in which a sample is selected from elements or members of a population through non-random methods.

non-symmetrical distribution (skewed distribution) Frequency distribution in which the distribution has an off-centre peak. If the tail of the distribution points to the right, the distribution is said to be positively skewed; if the tail of the distribution points to the left, the distribution is said to be negatively skewed.

normal curve A bell-shaped curve that graphically depicts a normally distributed frequency distribution. (*See* normal distribution.)

normal distribution A symmetrical, bell-shaped theoretical distribution; has one central peak or set of values in the middle of the distribution.

null hypothesis (HO) A statistical hypothesis that predicts that no relationship exists between variables; the hypothesis that is subjected to statistical analysis.

nursing research Research that focuses on developing knowledge of the care of persons in health and illness; generating knowledge of policies and systems that effectively and efficiently deliver nursing care; the profession and its historical development; ethical guidelines related to the delivery of nursing services; and systems that effectively prepare nurses to fulfil the profession's current and future social mandate.

O

observational research A data-collection method in which data are collected through visual observations.

open-ended questions Questions that allow respondents to answer in their own words.

operational definition The definition of a variable that identifies how the variable will be observed or measured.

ordinal level of measurement Data can be categorised and placed in order; small, medium and large is an example of a set of ordinal data.

P

parameter A numerical characteristic of a population; for example, the average educational level of people living in Gauteng province.

parametric tests A type of inferential statistic that is concerned with population parameters. When parametric tests are used, assumptions are made that (a) the level of measurement of the data is interval or ratio, (b) data are taken from the populations that are normally distributed on the variable that is being measured, and (c) data are taken from populations that have equal variances on the variable that is being measured.

participant observer – covert The research observer interacts with the participants and observes their behaviour without their knowledge.

participant observer – overt The research observer interacts with participants openly and with their full awareness.

percentage (%) A statistic that represents the proportion of a subgroup to a total group, expressed as a percentage ranging from zero to 100 per cent.

percentile A data point below which lies a certain percentage of the values in a frequency distribution.

personality inventories Self-report measures used to assess the differences through the descriptions of the meanings of these experiences provided by the people involved.

pilot study A small-scale trial run of an actual research study.

population A complete set of persons or objects that possess some common characteristic that is of interest to the researcher.

positively skewed A frequency distribution in which the tail of the distribution points to the right.

positive relationship (direct relationship) A relationship between two variables in which the variables tend to vary together; as the values of one variable increase, the values of the other variable increase.

predictive validity A type of criterion validity of an instrument in which a determination is made of the instrument's ability to predict the behaviour of participants in the future.

pre-existing data Existing information that has not been collected for research purposes.

pre-experimental design A type of experimental design in which the researcher has little control over the research situation; includes the one-shot case study and the one-group pre-test–post-test design.

primary source An account of a research study that is presented by the original researcher(s); in historical data, primary sources are those that provide first-hand information or direct evidence of an event.

probability sampling (including simple, stratified, cluster and systematic random sampling) The use of a random sampling procedure to select a sample from elements or members of a population.

probes Prompting questions that encourage the respondent to elaborate on the topic that is being discussed.

productive writing Writing reports on a regular basis, producing goal-directed reports.

projective technique A self-report measure in which a participant is asked to respond to stimuli that are designed to be ambiguous or to have no definite meaning. The responses reflect the internal feelings of the participant that are projected upon the external stimuli.

proposal A plan or suggestion, especially a formal or written one, put forward for consideration or discussion by others.

R

reliability The consistency and dependability of a research instrument in measuring a variable; types of reliability are stability, equivalence and internal consistency.

replication study A research study that repeats or duplicates an earlier research study, with all the essential elements of the original study held intact. A different sample or setting may be used.

research design The overall plan for gathering data in a research study.

research hypothesis (H1) (scientific, substantive or theoretical hypothesis) An alternative hypothesis to the statistical null hypothesis; predicts the researcher's actual expectations about the outcome of a study.

research instruments (research tools) Devices used to collect data in research studies.

research report A written or oral summary of a research study.

retrospective studies Studies in which the dependent variable is identified in the present (for example, a disease condition) and an attempt is made to determine the independent variable (for example, cause of the disease) that occurred in the past.

rows Horizontal entries in a table.

S

sample A subset of the population that is selected to represent the population.

sampling bias (1) The difference between sample data and population data that can be attributed to a faulty selection process; (2) a threat to the external validity of a research study that occurs when participants are not randomly selected from the population.

sampling distribution A theoretical frequency distribution that is based on an infinite number of samples. Sampling distributions are based on mathematical formulas and logic.

sampling error Random fluctuations in data that occur when a sample is selected to represent a population.

sampling frame A listing of all the elements of the population from which a sample is to be chosen.

scatter plot (scatter diagram, scattergram) A graphic presentation of the relationship between two variables. The graph contains variables plotted on an X axis and a Y axis. Pairs of scores are plotted by the placement of dots to indicate where each pair of Xs and Ys intersect.

secondary sources An account, in the research literature, of a research study that is written by someone other than the study investigators; in historical data, secondary sources and second-hand information or data are provided by someone who did not observe the event.

selection bias A threat to the internal validity of an experimental research study that occurs when study results are attributed to the experimental treatment when, in fact, the results may be due to

pre-treatment differences between the participants in the experimental and comparison groups.

semantic differential An attitude scale that asks participants to indicate their position or attitude about some concept along a continuum between two adjectives or phrases that are presented in relation to the concept that is being measured.

skew A frequency distribution that is non-symmetrical.

snowball sampling A sampling method that involves the assistance of study participants to help obtain other potential participants.

standard deviation (SD) A measure of variability; the statistic that indicates the average deviation or variation of all the values in a set of data from the mean value of that data.

standard error of the mean (sx) The standard deviation of the sampling distribution of the mean.

structured interviews The interviews ask the same questions in the same manner of all respondents.

survey studies Research studies in which self-report data are collected from a sample in order to determine the characteristics of a population.

symmetrical distributions Frequency distributions in which both halves of the distribution are the same.

systematic review A systematic review is formal research that follows systematic methods and a predefined structure to find and appraise research studies focusing on answering a similar question. The results of a systematic review synthesise studies and could provide a reliable picture of what is known and what remains uncertain.

T

theoretical framework A study framework based on prepositional statements from a theory of theories.

theory A set of related statements that describes or explains phenomena in a systematic way.

time sampling Observations of events or behaviours that are made during certain specified time periods.

triangulation The use of multiple methods or perspectives to collect and interpret data about some phenomenon; to converge on an accurate representation of reality.

U

univariate study A research study in which only one variable is examined.

unstructured interviews The interviewer is given a great deal of freedom to direct the course of the interview; the interviewer's main goal is to encourage the respondent to talk freely about the topic that is being explored.

unstructured observations The researcher describes behaviours as they are viewed, with no preconceived ideas of what will be seen.

V

validity The ability of an instrument to measure the variable that it is intended to measure.

variable A characteristic or attribute of a person or object that differs among the persons or objects that are being studied, for example, age or blood type.

volunteers Participants who have offered to participate in a study.

Index

Please note: Page numbers in *italics* refer to figures, diagrams or tables

A

abductive reasoning 134
accessible population 140, 141, 152
accidental sampling *see* convenience sampling
adequacy
    referral 185
    of sample 155
    scientific 208
all-inclusive sampling 141
analysis
    meaning of 191
    and philosophical inquiry 128, 129
    of qualitative data 135, *135*, 206
    of quantitative data 135, *135*, 192–193
    secondary 173
    strategies for 191–192
    techniques 55, 126
    triangulation 102
    see also data analysis
ANOVA 204
applied research 10, 103, 194
appropriateness
    of data-collection instrument 187
    of research problem 63
    of research tools 24
argumentation, and philosophical research 129
ascertainment bias 142
assisted death/dying 33, 64
associative hypothesis 88, *88*
authenticity, and credibility of data 186
authorities, and knowledge acquisition 5–6
availability sampling *see* convenience sampling

B

basic research 10, 102–103
bias
    and external validity 113
    and quantitative research 9, 101
    sampling 142–143
    in selection 110, 112, 142

C

categorising, and qualitative data analysis 207
causal hypothesis 88, *88*, 89, *89*
cause–effect relationship 109, 111, 203
census, and sampling 119, 141
central tendency, measures of 198, *198*
chance factor, in sampling 142
clinical trials 10, 16, 109
    see also randomised control trials
closed-ended questions 165, *165–166*, 166
cluster sampling 147–148
coding, and qualitative data analysis 207
coercion, and ethical principles 35–36
communication
    and informed consent 42
    online 127
    and qualitative data 207
    phase, of research process 50, 55–56
    technologies 45
    trends 168
comparative descriptive study 115
comparison group 110
complex hypotheses 89, *89*
computer programs, and qualitative data
    analysis 208
concealment, and ethical principles 36
concepts 28, 29, *29*
conceptual
    framework 20, 21, 26–27, 52, 70
    phase, of research process 51–53
concurrent validity 179–180
confidentiality
    agreement 43
    breaches 39
    and informed consent 40, *41*
    procedures 38, 39
confirmability, and trustworthiness 130, 131,
    132, 184, 185
consecutive sampling 152
consent
    and assent 42

and children 42
and choice 42
and deception 43
form/letter 40, *41*, 42, 45
and information 39
and online data 209
and research ethics 34
and research ethics committees (RECs) 4
and researchers 42, 43
and understanding 42
see also informed consent
constructs 28, 29, *29*
construct validity 180–181
content validity, and data collection 177–178
context, in qualitative research 123, 132
contingency tables 202, 203, *203*
continuous errors *see* systematic errors
contrasted groups 180
control
    group *105*, 107–108, 110, 195, *195*
    and randomised control trials 109
convenience sampling 149–150
convergence, validity from 180
correlation coefficients, types of 201–202, *201*
correlational designs 11, 116, 117, *133*
Covid-19
    and acquiring knowledge 6
    and ethics 33
    and online learning 67
    and phenomenological research 125
credibility
    definition of 130, 184
    and dependability 185
    techniques to achieve 130–131, 185
    and trustworthiness 183, 184
criterion-related validity, and data collection
    178–180
critical incidents (data collection technique) 173
critical
    realism 25
    review 78
    theory 23, 25
crossover design, and randomised control
    trials 109
cross-sectional study 103–104, 105, 116, 118
cross-tabulation table 202, *203*

D
data
    cleaning 206
    enhancement strategies 186–187
    management, and qualitative data
        analysis 206
    protection, and online research 209
    quality 186–187
    saturation 151, 153, 185, 186
    type of 53, 55, 57, 205
    triangulation 102, 130, 132, 134
data analysis
    approach to 55
    and descriptive statistics 193–203
    evaluation 208–209
    and graphics 205, 209
    and inferential statistics 203–205
    and online research 209
    in qualitative research 206–208
    plan 53
    strategies for 191–192
    see also analysis
database(s) 74, 75, 76
data collection
    and consent 39, 40
    context/setting 160
    definition of 157
    errors in 101
    and ethical principles 36, 46
    and interviews 169–171
    methods/techniques 54, 123, 125–127,
        160–173, *163–164*, *165–166*
    planning of 158–160
    and research design 53, 54, *135*, 135–136
    and sample size 154
data-collection instruments
    and data quality 186–187
    and observation 160–162
    and pre-test 54, 131, 188
    reliability of 181–183
    and research design 53
    and sample size 154
    self-support 163–172, *163–164*, *165–166*, *171*
    types of 159–160
    validity of 177–181
deception
    and ethical principles 36

and informed consent 43
deductive reasoning 6, 7, 134, 207
delimitations, and sampling 140
dependability, and credibility of data 185
dependent variable(s) 89, *89*, 90, 91–92, 110, 116
descriptive
    codes, and qualitative data analysis 207
    correlational designs 11, 116
    data, and observation 160, 161
    designs 11, 114–116
    epidemiology 118
    research design 191–192
    studies 11, 104, 115
descriptive statistics
    definition of 192, 193
    and frequency distributions 193–198
    and level of measurement 194–196, *194*,
        195, *196*
    simple 196–203
directional hypothesis 88
disproportionate stratified sampling 147
distinguishing descriptors 140
divergence, validity from 180
double-blind procedure, and randomised control
    trials 109

E
effect size, and randomised control trials 109
efficiency, of data-collection instrument 187
electronic questionnaires 168–169
eligibility criteria 140
empirical
    literature 123
    phase, of research process 54
    questions 86
    testing 87
environmental factors, in measurement
    errors 177
epidemiological
    data 119
    process 118–119
    research 117
    studies, uses in health sciences of 118
    triad 117
epidemiology
    categories of 118
    definition of 117
    purpose of 118

epistemology 23, 26
equivalence reliability, of research
    instrument 182–183
error
    in data collection 101
    in measurement
    sources of 176–177
    types of 175–176
ethical
    analysis 129
    clearance 54
    guidelines 46, 47
    review(s) 45
ethical research
    and anonymity 38
    codes of 34–35
    and coercion 35, 36
    and confidentiality 38, 39
    and full disclosure 36
    guidelines in 35, 43, 67
    and indigenous people/communities 34
    and privacy 38
    and self-determination 35
ethics
    committees 40, 43, 45–46
    review boards 45–46
ethnographic researchers 71
ethnography
    and analysis 126
    and data collection 126
    definition of 126
    derivatives 126
    forms of 126
    and online research 127
    in phenomenological studies 124
event sampling 161, 162
evidence-based
    decision-making process 14
    information 214–215
    medicine (EBM) 14
    practice (EBP) 5, 12, 13–14, 15
evidence-informed care 4
exclusion criteria, for sampling 140
experimental
    designs 105–109, 111, *105–106*, 162
    epidemiology 118
    group 107–108, 194, 195, *195*
    intervention 108, 110, 111, 112

research 10, 92
explanatory
    design 134, 136
    mixed methods design 71
    sequential mixed methods 135, *135*
    studies 104
exploratory
    design 134, 135, 136
    mixed methods design 71
    questions 86
    research 169
    sequential mixed methods 135, *135*
    studies 166
extraneous variable(s) 57, 92, 106

F

face validity, and data collection 177
factorial designs *105*, 109
feasibility, and research problem 64, 65
field notes
    and data analysis 206–207
    and ethnography 126
    and observation 161, 170
focus group interviews 170
foundational studies 129
framework, of research study 20, 21, 26–27, 52, 70
frequency distributions (in statistics) 193–196, *194*, *195*, *196*

G

generalisability, of data-collection instrument 187
golden thread 67–68
grand theory 21, *21*, 22
graphics
    and data analysis evaluation 209
    use of *200*, 205
grounded theory
    description of 127
        and data collection 127–128
    and basic social processes (BSPs) 128
    and theoretical sampling 151
        and qualitative research 71

H

Hawthorne effect 113, 176
Helsinki, Declaration of 34–35
hermeneutic sciences 25
hermeneutic-phenomenological sciences 25
homogeneity *see* internal consistency
hypotheses
    characteristics of operational 87
    definition of 86–87
    testing of 30, 87
    types of 88–89, *88*, *89*

I

implied consent 39, 40
inadequate design 101, 202
inclusion criteria, for sampling 140, 187
independent variable(s) 89, *89*, 90, 91, 109, 110, 116
inductive reasoning 6, 134
inferential statistics 115, 192–193, 203–205
informed consent
    and children 42
    elements of 39–42
    form/letter 40–41, *41*, 42
    guidelines regarding 43
    and online data 209
    and research committees 40
    see also consent
inquiry audits, and credibility of data 185
institutional review boards (IRBs) 45
instruments *see under* data collection
instrumentation
    and internal validity 112
    and measurement errors 176, 177
intention-to-treat analysis, and randomised control trials 109
internal consistency, of research instrument 182
interpretation(s)
    evaluation of 80
    and grounded theory 127, 128
    and information/sources 72, 73
    and paradigms 24
    and phenomenological research 124
    and philosophical enquiry 129
    of qualitative data 206, 207, 208
    of quantitative data 192, 194
    and quantitative research 99, 100
    and research design *135*

and research reports 213, 214
of results 55
and search strategy 74
and trustworthiness 130, 131, 184, 185
interpretive phase/stage, of research process
   50, 55
interpretivism 23, 25, 134
inter-related reliability 183
interval
   data 171, 192, 195–196, *195, 196*, 198, 199
   sampling 146, *146*
   scales 159, *201*, 204,
intervention
   experimental 108, 110, 111, 112
   protocol, and randomised control trials 109
interviewers
   role and influence of *164*, 169, 171
   training of *164*, 170
interviews
   strengths and weaknesses *163–164*
   types of 169–170

J

judgemental sampling *see* purposive sampling

K

knowledge acquisition
   alternative methods of *8–9*
   scientific method of 4, 8, *8–9*
knowledge translation 50, 56, 103

L

Likert scale 171–172, *171*
literature review
   definition of 69–70
   evaluation of 80
   guidelines for writing of 79–80
   information to include in 72–73
   and mixed methods research 134
   outline for 78
   process 76–78
   purpose of 52, 69, 70–71
   in qualitative research 71, 123
   in quantitative research 71
   and research reports 217
   and search strategy 74–76
   types of 70

longitudinal
   design 11, 115, 116
   research 104
   study 42, 103, 104, 115

M

manual analysis, and qualitative data 207
maturation 103, 108, 112
mean
   calculation of 198, 200, 201
   definition of 198, 199
measurement evaluation, checklist for 188–189
median 198, 200
member checks, and credibility 184
meta-analysis 16, 70, 71, *105*, 118
metaparadigm 25
metatheory 20, *21*
methodological triangulation 102
methodology 16, 23
micro-theory 22
middle-range theories 21–22, *21*
mixed methods
   design 4, 71, 134–136, *135*
   studies 71
mixed methods research 4, 24, 25, 122
   definitions of 133–134
   and pragmatism 134
   and sample choice 152
mode 198, 199, 200
model(s), in health sciences 26, 27, 49, 56, 57
mortality 111, 112, 118, 119
motivation
   and predictive validity 179
   and productive writing 223, 224
   and research problem 66, 67
   theory *62*
multi-centred RCTs 109
multistage sampling 148
multi-trait, multi-method approach, and
   construct validity 180–181

N

narrative, and data analysis evaluation 209
narrow-range theory 22
National Health Act (61 of 2003) 35, 47
National Health Research Ethics Council
   (NHREC) 35

naturalistic setting 57, 106
negative case analysis 131, 185
nested approach (and sample choice) 152
nominal
     data 194, *194*, 198, 202, 205
     scales 158, *201*
non-directional hypothesis 88
non-empirical questions 85
non-equivalent control group design 110
non-experimental designs 105, *105–106*,
     113–114, 162
     categories of 114–117
non-experimental research/approach 10, 11, 105
non-parametric statistics 204–205
non-probability sampling
     description of 148–149
     disadvantages of 148–149
     and online research 149
     and representativeness 148
     techniques/types of 148, 149–152
non-response error, in sampling 142
non-traditional designs *105*, 132
normal
     curve, definition of 199
     distribution, definition of 199, 200, *200*
null hypothesis 89
Nuremberg Code 34, 35

O
observation
     advantages and disadvantages of 162
     critiquing of 162
     definition of 160
     timing of 161–162
     types of 161
observational methods, guidelines to 162
online
     communication 127
     interviews 171
     learning 67, 127
     questionnaire 163, 168
     techniques, and random sampling 144
online data
     collection 160, 163, 170, 206
     and consent and permissions 209
     protection of 209
online research
     and ethics 33, 34, 45

     and field notes 206
     and non-probability sampling 149
     and protection of data 209
     and scientific theory 20
ontology 23, 26
open-ended questions 165, 166
operational hypotheses, characteristics of 86
opinion(s)
     and authorities 5, 6
     and hierarchy of evidence 16
     and interviews 170
     and literature review 72, 73
     variables 115
ordinal
     data 194–195, *195*
     scales 158–159, 205

P
paradigms
     assumptions of 23
     definition of 23, 24
     groups of 24–25
     see also metaparadigms
paradigmatic approaches relevant to science 23
parameter, definition of 141
parametric statistics 203–204
partially controlled setting(s) 57
participant(s)
     availability 64, 65, 66
     and beneficence 37
     and bias 101, 142
     and ethical research guidelines 35, 36
     and ethnography 126
     and experimental design 10, 107, 109
     and external validity 113
     factors in measurement errors 176–177
     and grounded theory 127
     human rights of 34, 35, 36, 37
     and informed consent 39–43, *41*
     and internal validity 111, 112
     and justice 38–39
     and non-probability sampling 148, 149
     online recruiting of 149
     and potential benefits and risks 44
     and probability/random sampling 143,
          144, 145
peer debriefing 130, 184
persistent observation, and credibility 184

phenomenological research/study 53, 71, 124–126
philosophical
   analysis 63, 129
   inquiry 128, 129
philosophy 23, 26, 128, 129
physiological measures, of data collection 170
pilot study 54, 187–188
population (in study)
   definition of 53, 140
   and elements of sample 141
   and inclusion criteria 140
   and non-probability sampling 148, 149, 150, 151
   parameter 114, 141
   and probability sampling 143, 144, 145, 146
   representativeness of 141–142
   and research design 53, 114
   statistics 119
   see also sample
positivism 23, 25, 134
post-test-only control group design *105*, 108, 109, 194
practice theory 20, *21*, 22
pragmatism 134
predictive validity 179
preliminary phase 78
preliminary study *see* pilot study
pre-test 54, 107, 112, 187–188
pre-test–post-test control group design 107, 108
probability sampling
   in quantitative studies 153
   and sample adequacy 155
   and sampling error 142
   techniques 143, 146, 148
   see also random sampling
problem statement 60, 67, 87
process consent 39, 42
productive writing 223–224
prolonged engagement, and credibility 184
proposition 28–29, *29*
prospective
   designs 11
   studies 104, 105, 117
purpose statement 67, 84
purposive samples/sampling 148, 150–151, 153, 185–186

Q
qualitative
   data 55, 134–136, *135*, 206–208
   design 133–136, *135*
   reliability, definition of 184
   studies, and sample size 153
   validity, definition of 183
qualitative research
   and beneficence 37
   key features of 122–123
   and literature review 71, 123
   methods, and validity 181
   and philosophical inquiry 128, 129
   principles of 3
   and rigour 129
   and scientific method 9
   and trustworthiness 130, 131, 132
quantitative
   epidemiology 118
   studies 153, 219
quantitative data
   analysis of 55, 192–193
   interpretation of 206
   and mixed methods research 133–136, *135*
   organising of 191
quantitative research
   and bias 101
   and causality 100
   literature review in 71
   principles of 3
   and probability 101
   and rigour 100
   and scientific method 9, 53, 87
quantitative research design
   classification of 105–106, *105–106*
   concepts and principles in 100–102
   and epidemiological research 117–119
   evaluation of 119
   experimental designs 106–113
   non-experimental designs 113–117
quasi-experimental
   designs 87, *106*, 110
   research 10, 92
questionnaires
   development of 164, 178
   distribution of 168–169
   electronic 168–169
   qualities of well-designed 163

reviewing of 168
strengths and weaknesses of *163–164*
questions (in questionnaires)
arrangement of 167–168
construction of 165–168, *165–166*
formulation of 166–167
quota sampling 148, 150
quotations, and review report 79

R

random
assignment, vs random sampling 107
errors, in measurement 175–176
numbers, table of 144–145, *145*
sample stratified according to size 147, *147*
selection 112, 143, 144
random sampling
using Excel 144
vs random assignment (randomisation) 107
and randomised control trials 109
simple 143–146, *145*
stratified 146–148, *146, 147*
see also probability sampling
randomisation 10, 107, 108, 109, 110
randomised control trials (RCT) 16, 17, 109
range, definition of 199
ratio
data 195–196, *195, 196*
scales 159
reactive effects 113
recorded consent 39
recording information 77
records, as source of information 172–173
referral adequacy, and credibility 185
reflexivity, and credibility of data 185
relationship, measures of 201–203, *201, 202, 203*
relevance of data 75, 130–131
reliability
definition of 181
of data-collection instruments 181–183
and relationship with validity 183–186
report
ethics of writing 2 22
evaluation of 222–223
formats 214
planning 214–216
structure of 216–220
style of 220–221

technical layout of 221–221
representative sample 141–142
representativeness, of sample/population 6, 132, 141–142, 147, 148
research
aims/objective(s) of 60, 85, 90, 139
approach 53, 55
categories of 3–4
characteristics of 2–3
definitions of 3–4
design, choice of 132–133, *133, 135*
ethics committees (RECs) 40, 43, 45, 94
hypothesis 52, 89, *154*
idea development 61, *61–63*
integrity 45
method 52, 53, 55
participants 38–44, 54
phases/stages 49–50
proposal(s) 45, 46, 54, 94–96
traditions, dominant 25
research findings
application/implementation of 13, 39, 103
communicating of 56
dissemination of 213
evaluation of 12
and literature review 72
reliability and validity of 129
research problem
appropriateness of 63
considerations regarding 63–66
definition of 51, 59, 60
elements of 66–67
guidelines for formation of 67
identification of 51, 52
and literature review 70
and online learning 67
and participant availability 65–66
and researcher expertise 66
sources of 61–63, *61–63*
research process
communication phase of 55–56
conceptual phase of 51–53
empirical phase of 54
interpretive stage of 55
phases/stages of 49–50
steps in 50, *50*
research reports
aim of 214

elements of 213
ethics of writing 222
evaluation of 222–223
formats of 214
planning of 214–216
structure of 216–217–220
style of 220–221
technical layout of 221
researcher
    and 'basic social processes' (BSPs) 128
    effects 113, 132
    expertise 66
    factors, in measurement errors 177
    in grounded theory 127, 128
    in phenomenological studies 124
    in qualitative research 127, 128, 130
    subjectivity 101
    triangulation 102
result(s)
    in communication phase 56
    and hierarchy of evidence 15, 16
    in interpretative phase 55
    and mixed methods designs 135
    through applied research 103
retrospective design 11, 105, 116
review boards, role of 45–46

S

sample
    adequacy, and probability sampling 155
    choice 152
    definition of 140
    elements of 141
    imbalances 101
    population, representativeness of 6, 132,
        141–142, 147, 148
    statistics 141
    see also population
sample size
    determination of 154–155
    factors influencing choice of 153–154, *154*
    and sampling error 153
    selection of 152–153
sampling
    approaches 143–152
    bias 142–143
    definition of 139
    elements 140–141

error 142, 153
frame 141
and inclusion criteria 140
interval, calculation of 146, *146*
see also probability sampling; random
    sampling
scales (data collection instruments) *171*,
    171–172
scattergrams 202, *202*
scientific
    adequacy, and data analysis evaluation 209
    method 8–11, *8–9*
    observation 162
    research, definition of 2–3
search resources, types of 75
secondary analysis, definition of 173
self-determination, right to 35, 36, 42
self-report instruments/techniques
    definition of 162–163
    types of 163–172
semi-structured interviews 170
sensitivity, of data-collection instrument 186
significance 63
simple
    descriptive statistics 196–198, *196, 197*
    hypothesis 88–89, *88*
    random sampling 143–145, *145*
snowball sampling 148, 151–152
Solomon four-group design *105*, 108, 112
sources, for literature review 73, 75, 77–79
specification matrix 164–165, *165*
split-half method 182
spreadsheets 191
stability, of research instrument 182
standard deviation 199
statistical strategies, and data analysis 192
statistics
    and data analysis 192
    sample 141
stepwise replications, and credibility of data 185
stratified random sampling 146–147, *147*
structured
    interviews 169, 170
    observation 161
systematic
    errors, in measurement 176
    sampling 146, *146*

T

target population 10, 84, 140, 141, 142, 155
test-retest reliability 182
theme, and qualitative data analysis 207–208
theoretical
      framework 20, 27, 114
      sampling 151
thick description, of data 132, 185, 186
theory, levels/types of 20–22, *21*
triangulation
      and credibility 184
      design 134, 136
      and trustworthiness 130, 132
      types of 102
true experimental designs 106–107
trustworthiness
      of research instrument 183–186
      of a study 131, 132
t-test 204
typical descriptive study 115

U

unstructured
      interviews 169
      observation 161

V

validity (of research instrument) 177–181
      and relationship with reliability 183–186
      strategies to ensure 183–184
variables
      and research setting 57
      and theory development 28, 29, *29*, 30
variability
      measures of 199–201, *200*
      numerical value of 199
variance
      analysis of 204
      definition of 199
verbal consent 39
vignettes 172
virtual ethnography 127
voluntary consent 42, 43

W

web-based surveys 168
websites 48
written consent 35, 39